THE CALISTHENICS QUEST

SUPERHERO CALISTHENICS TRAINING

WRITTEN BY
RAY SHONK

FORWARD BY DANNY KAVADLO

Foreword
By Danny Kavadlo

In my years as a health professional, I've been a personal trainer, a PT manager, an author, a blogger, a fitness model and even an international presenter. Suffice it to say, I've worn a lot of hats in this industry and I've met a lot of trainers!

Some of these trainers are more memorable than others. Some have impressed me while others have not. But every now and again a trainer comes along who just "gets it."

I'm not just talking about understanding the science of training like sets, reps, and human anatomy—I'm a strong believer that anyone can learn that. No, I'm referring to something larger. Love, passion, spirit and more.

What I'm speaking of is the ability to connect to people, to resonate and to change lives. Hell, maybe even change the world.

Ray Shonk is such a trainer.

Ray and I first connected over social media several years ago. Since then, Ray has been my student at Dragon Door's acclaimed Progressive Calisthenics Certification, my comrade as a lifelong advocate of bodyweight strength training, and ultimately, I'm proud to say, my friend.

Ray has the rare gift of being able to motivate and inspire, while never coming across as overbearing. He leaves the work to his students, while providing exactly what they need from him in terms of instruction. Nothing more, nothing less. He is a true expert of his craft.

So as you might imagine, when a copy of The Calisthenics Quest appeared across my desk, I couldn't wait to tear into it. I found Ray Shonk's writing to be informative yet friendly. It's comprehensive, yet casual. He explores serious concepts with simplicity and humor. For example, when discussing the notion of challenging yourself, Shonk simply states: "It is called a workout, not an easy out. None of this will happen overnight."

So honest, simple and true—but definitely not easy!

Whether Ray is exploring the roots of bodyweight training, sharing his own anecdotes, or explaining the details of step-by-step exercise progression, he delivers the goods on bodyweight training—and then some!

One of my favorite passages appears toward the end of the work, when Mr. Shonk discusses the character building virtues of working out. In his signature style, he explains the importance of focusing on form and quality of movement, rather than only shooting for high reps and letting the ego take over. This type of process-mindedness is at the very core of Ray's philosophy as a trainer, a martial artist and a man. No rush here.

As Ray himself says, "This is your journey, so enjoy it."

-Danny Kavadlo, 2017

Chapter 1

"No man has the right to be an amateur in the matter of physical training. It is a shame for a man to grow old without seeing the beauty and strength of which his body is capable." -Socrates 469-399 BC

So, you've decided to undertake the quest for a new, healthy you. It will be a long journey, but it will be well worth it. This entire program is taking a minimalist approach to fitness through calisthenics. What is calisthenics? Calisthenics is an exercise method using your own body weight to achieve bodily fitness and grace of movement. It's beautiful and powerful at the same time. You are about to tap into beauty and power that is all generated from yourself. Sounds rather bad ass, doesn't it? You will get to move your body in one unified movement, just like our ancestors dating way back to the great mammoth hunters.

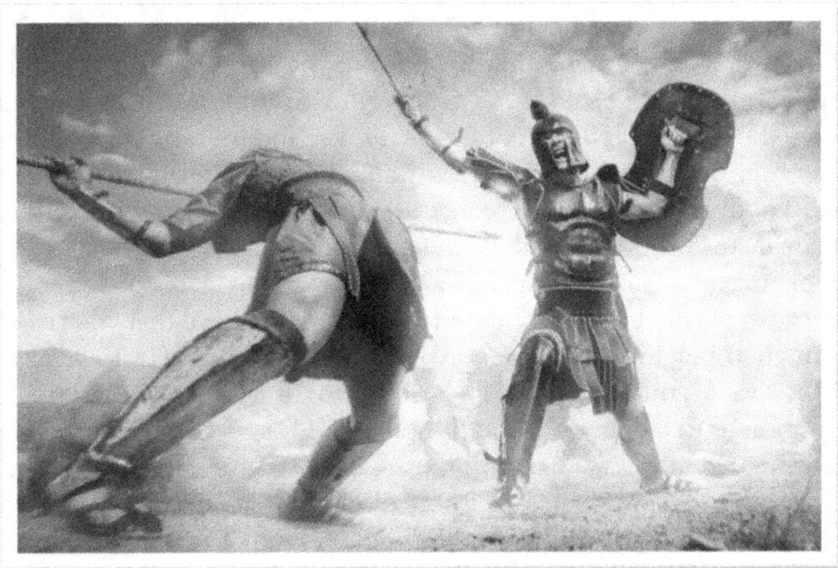

They didn't have big fancy gyms or fancy equipment. All they had was their hands. They climbed, jumped, ran and lived with the basics of push and pull. They had to do this if they wanted to survive. Imagine this: you wake up in your rocky cave and want to grab some breakfast. Well, you better chase it down, at the same time making sure you are not being chased down as something else's breakfast. With just our bodies we achieved great things.

Yes, back in ancient Greece they did have gyms, but nothing like we have today. It was almost all calisthenics based. Parallel bars, pull up bars, tracks. It was all they needed. Look at the old farmers before the days of big tractors! Those guys were a force of power. I remember seeing my grandpa in his older years lifting 4 bales of hay at once. Keep in mind each one of those weighs about 70 pounds! That's some epic strength for an 80-year-old man! Or even my calisthenics hero Jack Lalanne! He was amazingly strong even into his 90's. Let's look at the gym classes in the early 1900s. All you would see is jungle gyms, monkey bars, pull-up bars, Olympic rings and other calisthenics equipment. Yet, those guys were ripped and functionally strong! They never used a sit up machine, or a Lat pull down machine. What I'm trying to say is, since our start, fitness was woven into the very fabric of who we are, but the modern person hasn't unlocked this, yet...

Sadly, in a lot of schools, gym class has become a place to merely learn about sports, and not so much about getting healthy or fit. I think when I was in school, we had maybe one or two weeks of a strength training classes. Not nearly enough time to get fit or really learn the basics. Hell, we couldn't even use the fitness center without a teacher present, and none really wanted to stay after school for that. Most of my fitness in those years came from climbing trees or running through the woods, possible even reenacting scenes from a certain book that was about bringing a certain ring to a certain volcano. Because of situations like this, a lot of people believe that you need a gym membership at some massive franchise loaded with a lot of distractions and machines that offer no functionality or a lot of equipment to achieve a more fit body, and for a long time I was one of those people, but that simply isn't true. You already possess the best equipment available, your body. With this "equipment", you can become stronger, faster and more agile. Hell, I have gone outside and used a tree for pull-ups. The fresh air was a lot nicer than the smell of a sweaty gym. Know what is really nice? Going to a local park, back yard and your living room, requires no membership fee. For me, working out at the park makes me feel like a kid again. Is this the be all end all approach to fitness? No, there is no perfect workout that fits everyone. This is just one of many avenues of fitness. To be perfectly honest, if I had to choose a person that could nail one arm push-ups or the guy that could bench 200 pounds for my zombie survival team, I would pick the guy that could rock the push-ups. Keep in mind, no program you ever find will be a 100% substitution for working with a great trainer. But, this can be a good guide to get you started. Another thing to keep in mind is, this book is not a complete guide to calisthenics, it has been done, this is going to give you a hero training view to fitness. There are hundreds of exercises out in the calisthenics universe. So, once you are ready feel free to explore the calisthenics world and see what is out there. So, with this "equipment", let's begin your epic quest.

Why calisthenics?

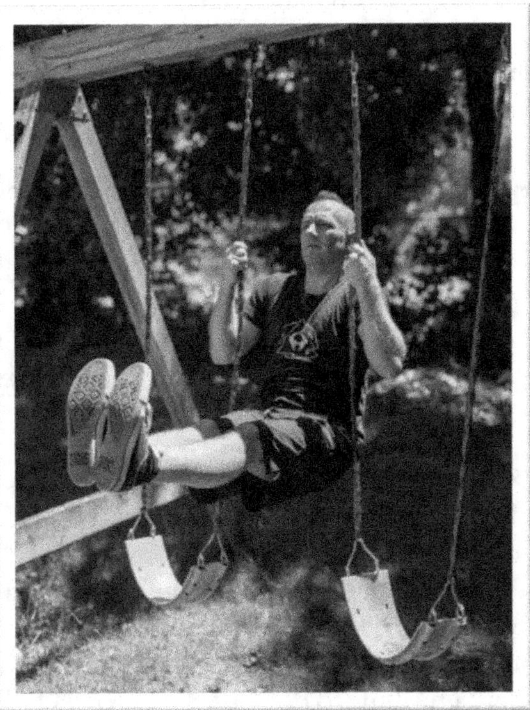

I have said this many times when training people and in fitness articles: there is nothing wrong with lifting weights. Matter of fact, I have a lot of friends and clients that prefer weights or one of the many other variations of fitness. That is 100% cool with me. They are getting their workout in. But for me I prefer to use my body. Calisthenics works multiple muscles at once and can constantly evolve around your current fitness level. With body weight training, it's always quality over quantity. Even better, you can do it almost anywhere! I love how calisthenics strengthens your muscles, sinew, bones and even your mind if you stay focused. It's a great way to become functionally fit. As soon as the form starts to fail, so too will the effect. Yes, I know not everyone can do a clean push-up or pull-up. In fact, most pull-ups I see in the gym are not "real" pull-ups. Don't worry! In this program, you will see the basic progressions for these kingly movements. With calisthenics you can hit your fitness goals if you stick to it. Here's the thing, once regular push-ups, pull-ups and squats get to easy, and they will, you level them up. That means increase the range of motion, change the style in which you do them or even change the tempo of the movement. The possibilities to level up your skill are near limitless. You get to choose how you want to advance the story! Everyone, including myself, loves a good superhero story, this is your chance to live one.

One question that I have asked in my calisthenics training and have been asked is, "Do I need to add weight to my calisthenics to get stronger?" The simple answer is no. Can you do it? Yes, but when I did some experimenting I found I could get just as strong by increasing the range of motion or playing with the tempo of the movement. In this book I will not be showing ways to add weight to your workouts, but you are welcome to experiment. Remember this is your fitness adventure. If you do add weight, then do so responsibly. Pay attention to your body and your form.

Remember: you are the hero in this quest and there will be obstacles with friends, family, work and everyday life. However, don't get discouraged; this is normal in every fitness journey. The important part is that you pick yourself up and continue on. I will tell you from experience life will happen, you will hit a point where you may want to give up. This is what separates the hero from the villager. You will do what others are unwilling to do. But, never forget to live, laugh and love. Make time for the work, but make time for your friends and family too. I will admit, it is so ingrained in me now that my wife insists I work out when I'm cranky. What's nice is a lot of my close friends have jumped into the calisthenics world. We will head out to local parks and all train together in large groups. We have almost become a local fitness tribe. Don't worry if you run into us out on the street, we always welcome newcomers. It's never a bad idea to have a few friends workout with you even if you are all different levels. My fit tribe keeps me motivated to keep working. No one in my group is the same level, but we all keep giving each other that little extra push to be the best we can be. This is one thing I have noticed in my time in the calisthenics world, we are one big brotherhood and sisterhood. It's not a competition, but a quest of self-betterment.

The Challenge!

You must always try to challenge yourself. If you want it to work, then you have to *work*. One thing I tell all my clients is, "It is called a *work*out, not an easy out. None of this will happen overnight." If you want to blow everyone away with push-ups, then you have to train them. None of this will be easy, and at first it will look impossible, but nothing in fitness is impossible if you work for it. I have personally watched people progress from never doing a push-up to nailing their first one arm push-up. Most important of all... Have fun with your workout! I personally like to make my workouts a game. I like to see if I can better my numbers from the week before or see if I can go deeper into a movement. Now, take a quick look in the mirror. That person you see is your only competition. Go ahead, take a picture of that person. With the right about of work and know how you will see a change. To be honest, I still have my picture of when I first started. You only need to strive to be better than you were yesterday. One thing I suggest is to schedule this into your day. Don't just wing it, plan the work and food. If you schedule it throughout the week you won't have to guess when you will fit it in. I will say this a few times in this program, it is better to get 30 – 40 minutes of hard focused work, than an hour and a half of doing half ass work. Put the phone down, ignore the random sports ball team on T.V. This is your time to slay the workout beast!

I say this to people over and over, there are no quick fixes in fitness! So many people want to find the easiest way to lose weight or get in better shape, but there isn't a cheat or magic elixir. I have seen fitness DVDs, nutrition shakes, diet plans and body wraps. Now let's think about this for a second. If there was one perfect quick way to lose weight or get fit, wouldn't that be the only one on the market? But they are everywhere! Here is the potion of truth, if you put in the proper work you will get the reward. Yes, it will take time, but in the end you can say you did it with no short cuts. The adventure is the best reward.

Progress or Regress?

Listening to your body is the key to progress. If it feels like you may be able to do one more push-up, then give it a shot, or maybe play with the hand or foot placement on those push-ups. Sometimes it's not about how many you can do, it can also be about how far you can push the range of motion. On the flip side of the coin, never be afraid to regress a movement if it feels like you are not getting quality from the movement. For example, if you can't get your arms to at least 90 degrees, then you may want to consider regressing the movement. Calisthenics is all about quality of the movement. I regularly regress my workouts just to get the most out of them. I even do this with my regular clients. Sometimes you have to take a step back so you can make a big leap forward. Most important is to leave your ego behind! It will only get in your way, and slow you down. Train smart! Yes, test your current limits, but don't force a movement. If you get injured this will be a major setback and lead to frustrations. One suggestion I will make is, if you want to get better at a movement such as push-ups, pull-ups or squats then train them more than once a week. Think about it, you didn't get good at walking by only doing it once a week. At the same time, you don't need to overdo it by training it every day. Throw in an extra set or two in through the week. Also, track your progress. Keep a fitness journal if anything just to remember what you did the last time you worked out. This is how you write your story of legends. As I said before, I also highly suggest taking a picture of yourself before you started this quest. This will be a constant reminder of how far you've come.

Another question I get from time to time is, "when should I add plyometrics into my workout?" This is a tricky one. First and foremost, ask yourself, "is my form top notch?" If it isn't quite there yet, hold off for a bit. Rushing off to battle before you properly train is foolhardy and the down fall of many heroes. If your form is doing great and you can knock out a bunch of reps of a move like push-ups then give it a try, but start small. Don't expect to do clapping push-ups on the first try. I would also suggest to put them in the beginning of your workout before you are too fatigued.

Chapter 2
Rest & Recover:

Hero! Your mana is low! A lot of my friends and clients that workout with me like to call me a machine, but I will tell you that even this machine needs his sleep. Everyone, regardless of their fitness level, needs rest. You could be the most bad ass fitness guru, and without rest your machine will start to fail. Rest is going to give your muscles time to repair themselves, so get plenty of sleep. I recommend 7-8 hours of sleep. All creatures in the animal kingdom need rest, and so do you. Keep in mind, if you are new to this extra activity, you will likely have no issue sleeping. My first night after fitness I think I slept like Rip Van Winkle. A good night's sleep will make you refreshed and ready for the next day's adventure.

In this time, your muscles will likely get sore. This normally happens within 24-48 hours. Staying slightly active in this time will help with the soreness. Also, make sure to drink plenty of water and eat quality foods. We will discuss foods shortly. To help with that Delayed Onset Muscle Soreness (DOMS), I like to take a nice hot shower or bath. On some occasions a nice massage or foam rolling my muscles really helps. Not only will I roll my muscles when sore, but I will also roll in my warm ups and cool downs. I'll go into foam rolling more in the warm ups and cool downs. Don't worry, the soreness is normal, you can still continue your workouts. If it is so horrible you can barely walk, then there is a good chance you pushed it a bit too hard. Never forget to listen to your body!

Active Rest:

You may have already noticed your quest includes active rest days. Active rest days are important to heal your body and, as you advance, you may not need as many. What is an active rest day? It is a day off of intense activity. I suggest going for a walk, a light bike ride, or even play with your kids in the park. Try to avoid just sitting on the couch playing video games and watching movies. For me, I like to do a lot of stretching or even martial arts training. I found the activity keeps me limber and fresh for the quest ahead. I wouldn't necessarily look at this as a day off, though many people treat it as such. I would look at it as the quiet before the storm. This is not an attempted to discourage you, but a warning that it can be incredibly easy to fall off the fitness path. It can honestly happen to anyone. Hell, I even fell off for a time. Remember the setbacks I mentioned before?

Warm Up Time:

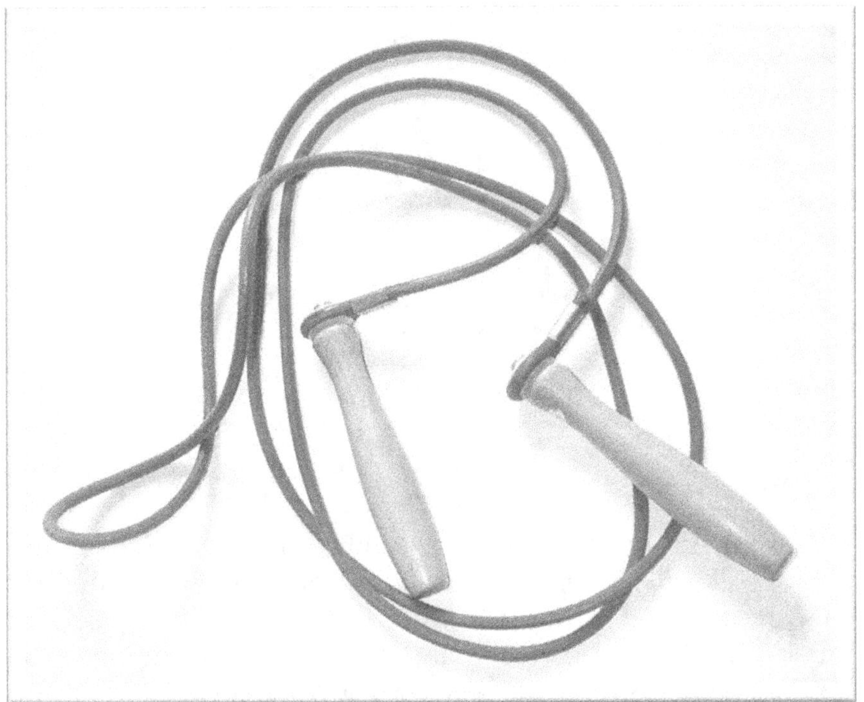

Before every workout, take 5 minutes to get in a quick warm up and stretch. This is going to help to prevent potential injuries. Remember, the workout is about results not injuries. I like to jump rope for my workout just to warm up my muscles, followed by an active stretch. Now my method may not be your method. Never forget we are all different levels and skill classes. Your ideal warm up may be a 5 min jog or a mile run. I even know people that will warm up with some interval training. If you are not sure what interval training is, don't worry, it will be covered. Again the important thing is that you warm up those muscles. Once your muscles are warm, get that good stretch in. Active stretching is a little different from your traditional stretch. These stretched you only hold for 1-3 seconds before you release tension. This will limber up the muscles without sacrificing that epic performance.

Cool Down:

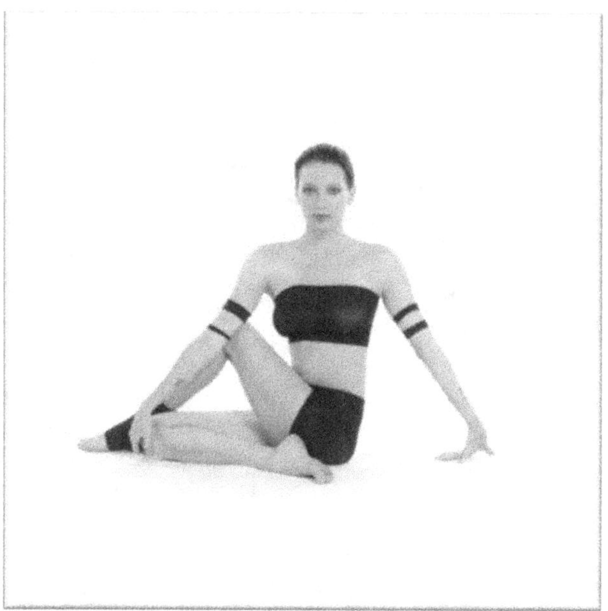

At the end of your daily journey, cool down your muscles. A light jog, fast walk and shaking out your limbs is a great way to cool down. I also recommend a nice static stretch or even a little yoga. Your muscles are warm right now and you can really improve your flexibility at this time. Take advantage of it. Static stretching is one that most people are familiar with. This is where you will hold the muscles at tension for 30 – 60 seconds. Once again, you need to listen to your body and know the limits of your stretch. You don't need to stretch so hard that you feel the dragon's fire in your muscle and tear your muscle. Take care of your fitness equipment!

Chapter 3

"Exercise is king. Nutrition is queen. Put them together and you've got a kingdom." -Jack Lalanne (AKA: The Godfather of Fitness)

Food:

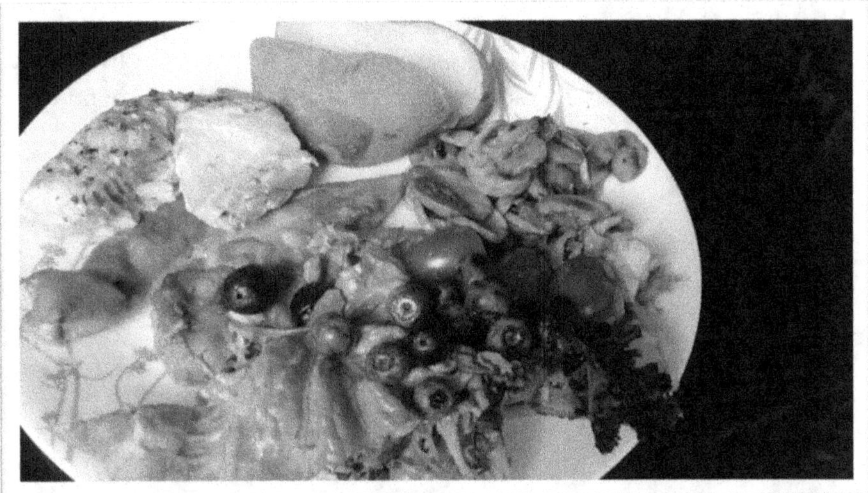

This is probably the most important part of your quest! Without food, we can't live. Everything living in this world needs sustenance. Try your best to not skip meals. The most important thing is to try to eat clean. Notice I said "try" ... No one is perfect, you may slip and that's ok. When I started out on my fitness journey, I was extremely strict on my diet. I will tell you, I was miserable! Then it backfired... I tried some of the foods I missed, and I binged. Afterwards, I felt like crap! After going through this cycle a few times, I realized to have a little fun from time to time. It will keep you from jumping off the fitness wagon and going insane with food lust. What I'm trying to say it, so what if you had a slice of pizza, have a nice salad to go with it, then pick yourself up and continue on. Even I have a cheat meal about every week, but I never lose sight of the goal. I'm guilty of being a beer and bourbon snob; hell, I even brew my own beer. With that said, when I do enjoy those drinks, I do so responsibly. I have maybe one beer or glass of bourbon and call it good. Also, if you are out on vacation don't be afraid to enjoy yourself a little. For example, when I took my first trip out to New York, I had to try New York pizza. Know what? I enjoyed the hell out of it! I even went out with a few friends and tried a burger I have never tried before, but for the side I went healthy over French fries and a large glass of water. Food can be your friend if you treat it right. But if abused, it can be an enemy to your fitness goal.

Things To Watch:

Stay away from ultra-low calorie diets, unless it is given to you by a medical professional. These programs tend to slow your metabolism and do not work long term. As a matter of fact, most people on these diets tend to gain all their weight back. These diets are not to be confused with fasting.

Also, watch out for those diets that tell you to cut all carbs or fats from your diet. Most people again don't fully read into these diets and end up with poor results in the long term. Carbs are your fuel. Take all the fuel out of your car and see how well it runs.

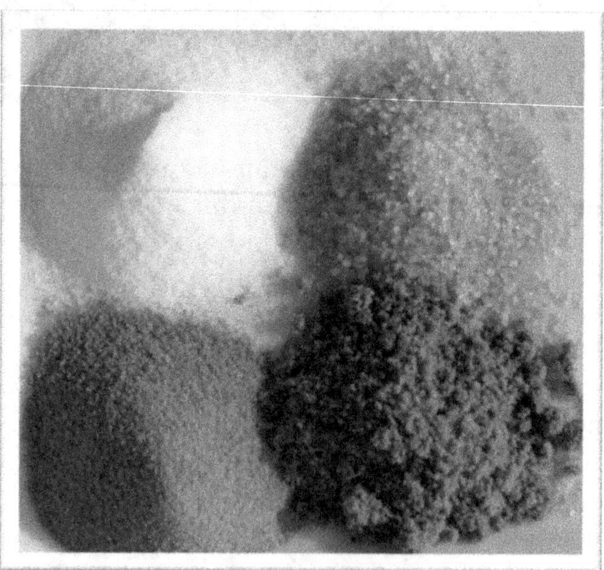

Ah sugar... It's hidden everywhere! It's the 6 pack assassin! The first thing I tell all my clients to try to ditch is the soda. Yes, even the zero calorie ones. The syrup it is made with is still some form of sweetener. Artificial sweeteners are not good for you and they should be avoided. Honestly even natural sweeteners should be avoided if possible. If you have that sweet tooth, like I do, try fruit instead. In time you will not miss those other sugars.

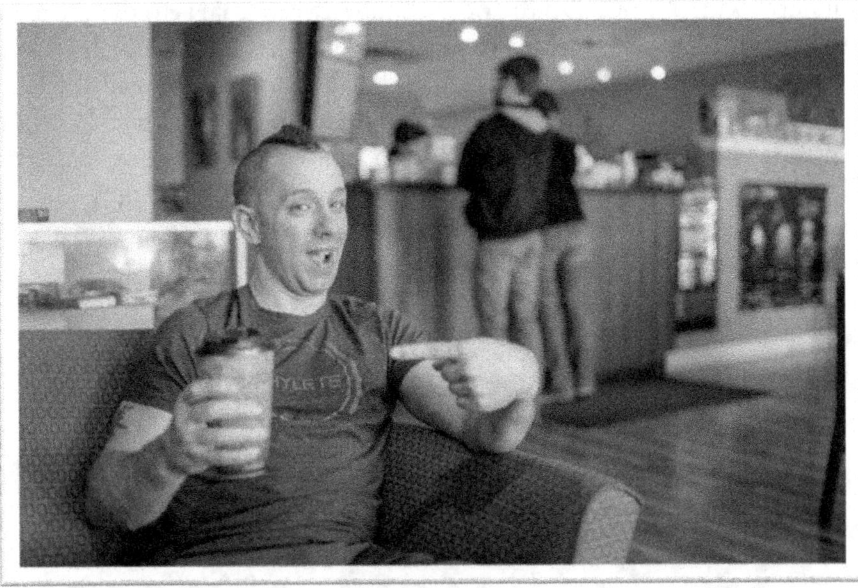

Coffee!!! I love coffee! If you need that boost for your day or for your workout, a cup of black coffee can hit the spot! But if it is just before a workout, be careful of the cream or milk you add. It could lead to a slightly upset stomach. A cup of coffee can also be a fantastic substitute for that chemical filled pre-workout drinks. Let's face it, we know the ingredients in coffee, ground coffee and water. But you never really know what is for sure in that energy drink. Also, believe it or not, research has shown there are health benefits to coffee including liver health. Ok, from time to time I like those fancy coffee drinks you get at fancy coffee shops, but remember what I said about sugar! They are more sugar now than coffee, twisted and evil. Well maybe not evil... can coffee have an alignment? Again, it is ok to indulge from time to time, but do so carefully. Because with great coffee, come great responsibility.

Calories in vs. Calories out or Quality of Food?

The answer is both. It's simple, if you want to gain weight, then you need to eat more calories than you burn, but not just high calorie foods, but instead good quality foods. Sure that fast food cheeseburger has the calories you need in a meal, but is it a good quality food? Nope! On the other hand, if your goal is to drop weight, then you need less calories than what you burn and you will have to also look at your ratio of protein, carbs and fats. As you will see later, you shouldn't cut any of these completely out of your diet. But both of these have to be done smart! Too many calories along with crap food will hide those new muscles under layers of fat, and too few calories may actually make you slow, sluggish and slow down your weight loss due to a slowing metabolism.

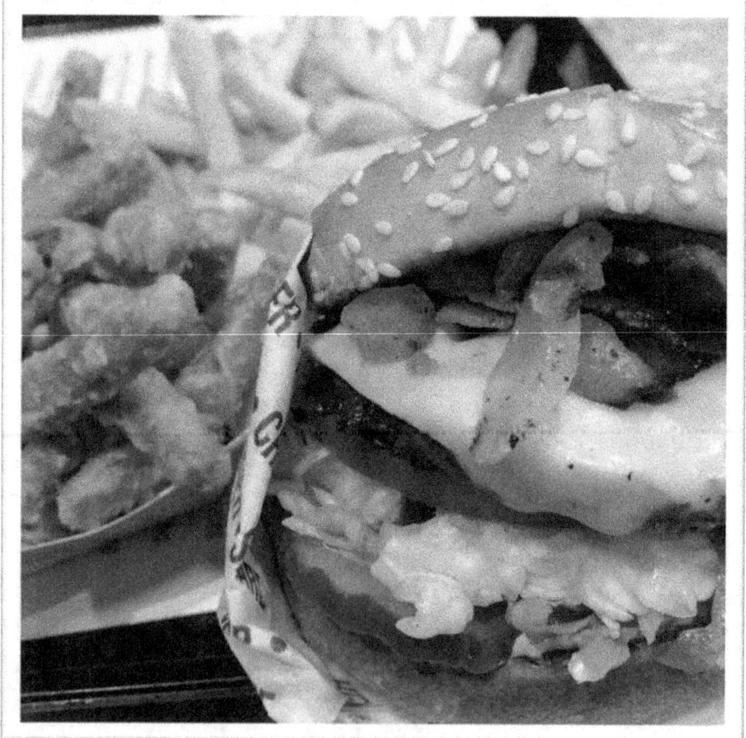

This can actually be common in the body building world. They do cuts to drop body fat, but doing this can cause metabolic damage, even though it is done for a short time. With calisthenics you will notice any weight gain. If you don't believe me then add 5 pounds to your push-up or pull-up. There are a lot of great apps available that can give you a good idea on how much you need based on height and weight. Remember, it won't be exact, everyone burns calories a little differently. No, you don't have to have chicken, brown rice, and broccoli at every meal. I've tried it, it's boring, and it really doesn't help the natural bacteria in your stomach to eat the same thing all the time. Don't punish the little happy bacteria, they help your belly. The human body craves variety, give it what it needs. Try to stick with foods that have as few ingredients as possible. Try to drop the box meals, and frozen dinners, they are full of junk your body really doesn't need. Keep it fresh, and lean.

Nutrition:

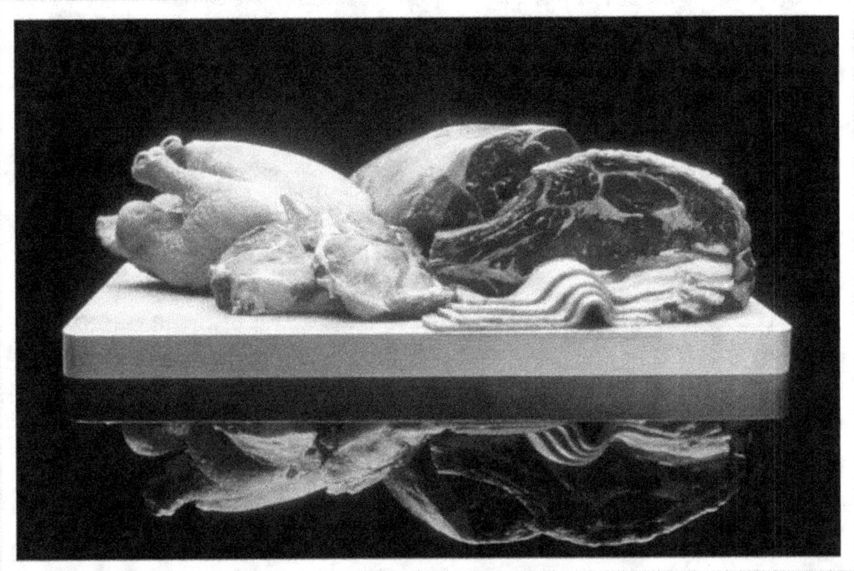

Proteins are important, but keep them lean. I'm sorry to say that greasy burgers probably isn't the best idea. Try to stick with lean proteins like tofu, salmon, tuna, chicken or lean red meats. You don't have to eat the same thing all the time. Try to have a little variety. Yes, I suggested tofu. I eat it regularly and I like it! Granted it doesn't really have a taste by itself, but you can make it taste like anything. It's not for everyone, but I say give it a go at least once. Eggs are also a great source of protein! Personally, I like to leave the yoke in. Yes, the yoke does have fat in it, but it also has a lot of great protein and nutrients that will do you good. Here is a common misconception about proteins, they are not actually an energy source. The proteins you eat actually help repair and rebuild muscle. Human muscles are made of meat! Don't eat people meat, it is wrong and will likely get you in lots of trouble. You would also likely be considered a weird zombie.

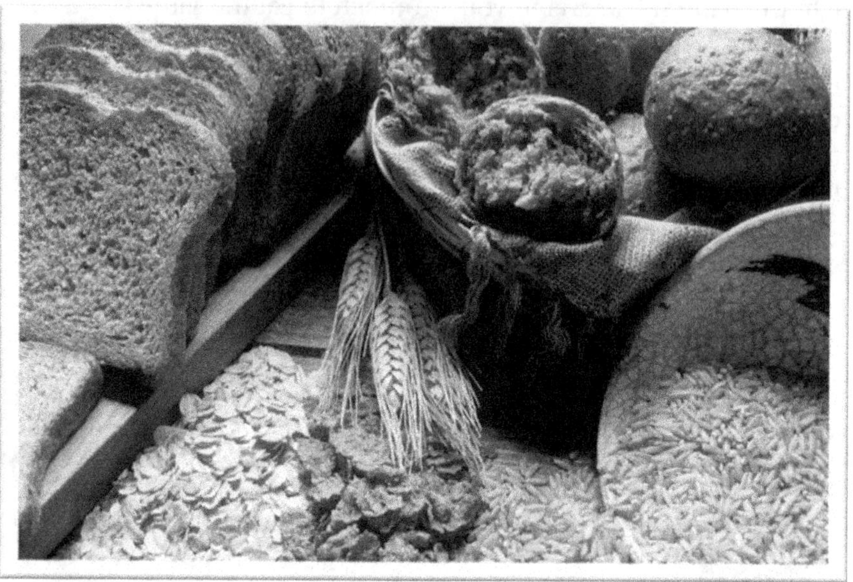

CARBS ARE IMPORTANT! So many diet and meal plans try to tell you that carbs are evil, but they are very important. Here is the truth: carbs are a fuel source for your body, but you have to do it right! Stay away from starchy carbs like french fries, white bread or even white rice. Your good carbs are things like sweet potatoes, brown rice, and other fruits and vegetables. Yes, fruits and vegetables are carbs, but you still need them. Again, try to have a variety on hand for meals and snacks. Don't just sit around eating bread and pasta all the time either! It is about proper portions of carbs. Yes, if you want to lose some body fat, you may have to reduce the carbs in your diet, but notice I said reduce, not cut out. Lowering your carbs will allow your body to use your body fat as a fuel source and in time lover your overall body fat content. If you still think you have to cut all carbs out of your diet, then try it and see how you feel. Odds are you will out of energy, maybe even a little cranky. I myself keep a steady flow of carbs in my system to keep my energy level up. Again, everyone's needs are different so this is something you can experiment with.

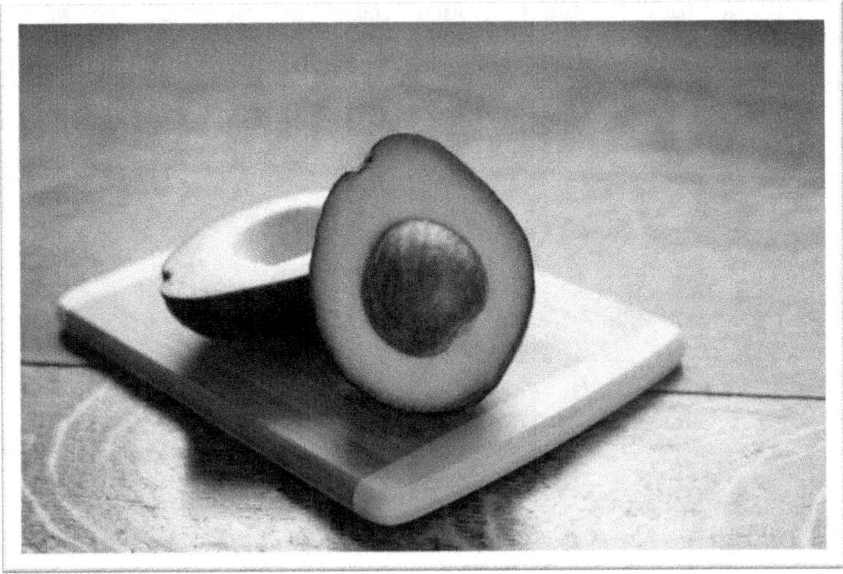

Fats are also important because you need them for proper brain and cell function. Believe it or not, fats are also a fuel source. But you need far less of them than you do carbs or proteins. No, not processed fats either. I'm talking good healthy fats like avocados, nuts, and natural oils like olive oil. Also, beware the foods labeled "low fat" or "no fat". Odds are it is a chemical shit storm, and it is better to have naturally occurring fats than the no fat chemicals that your body can't process. You have one life, explore a little, but do so responsibly.

Now onto supplements: You don't need them, despite what you are told at nutrition stores. You can get everything you need in the foods you eat, as long as you keep your diet balanced. Sure, you may see huge dudes at the gym tell you, you need "x amount" of protein before and after every workout or you have to cut all carbs from your diet to get the perfect results and you should stock up on this special supplement. I will admit I was one of those guys, I even sold supplements for a time. To be perfectly honest, your body can process only so much protein in one sitting. After that, you are just making expensive urine. After a lot of trial and error I realized, you don't need it! You should first know that no supplement is actually regulated by any governing body. Any random filler crap can be in there. I would rather enjoy a good meal on my fitness quest over drinking a random "magic" potion that I have no clue what the real ingredients are.

Chapter 4
Hollow the Body

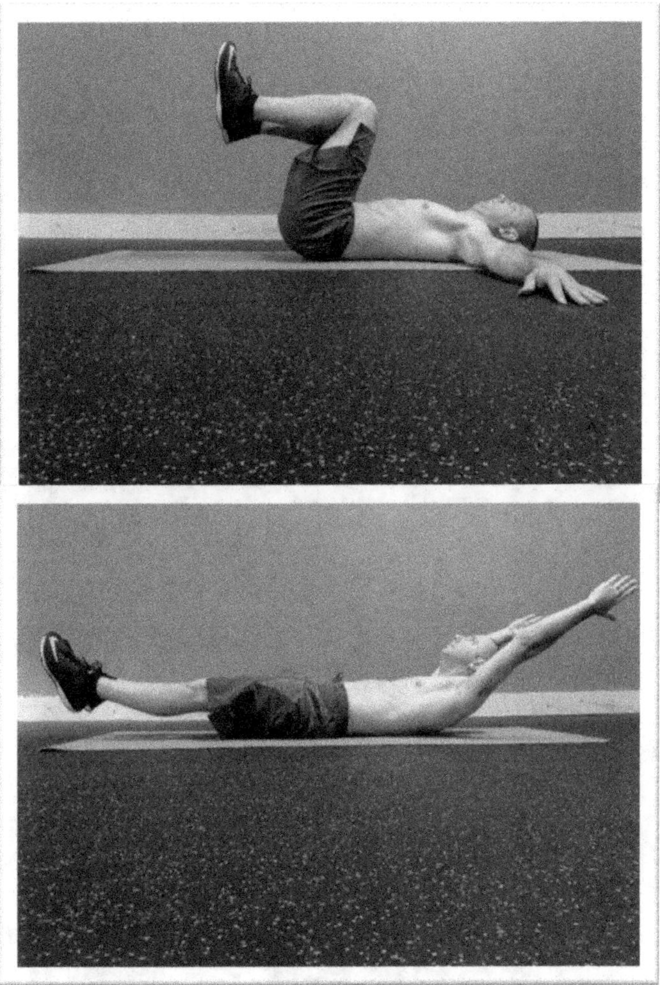

This training is great for learning to control your muscles. Many of my martial art students also refer to this as the "iron board". I suggest to train this often and to hold it as long as you can. To do this, start on the ground with your knees tucked into your chest, lower back pressed to the floor and arms resting at your side. Once in this position, slowly extend your legs out keeping your lower back pressed to the floor. Once you can get your legs fully extended and hold that, try tucking your chin and extending your arms over head. this is the full iron board. When you can hold this, your muscle control will show through and you will gain core strength. Become the iron board!

Cardio

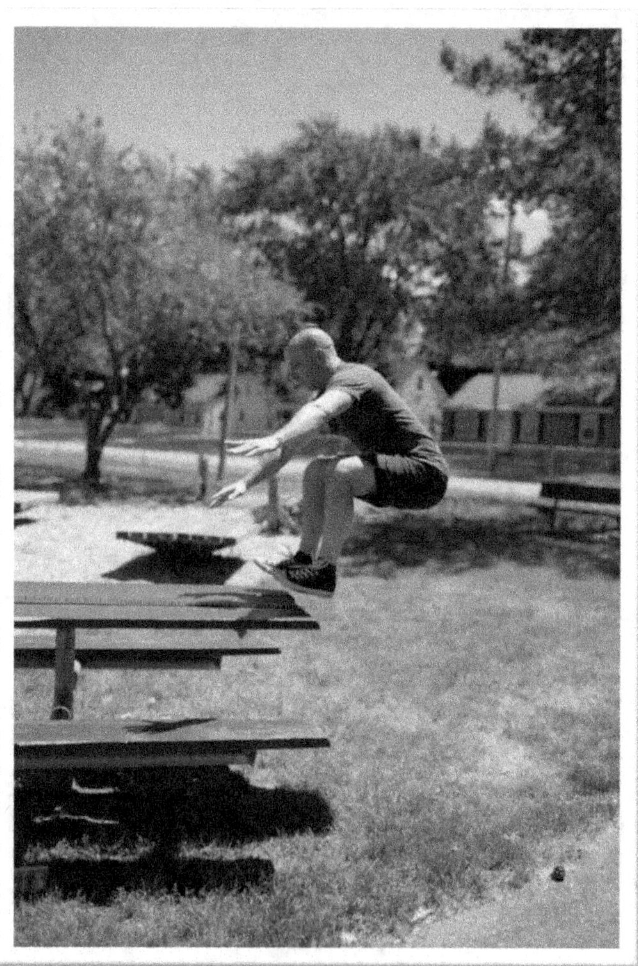

I'm rather sure cardio is the number one rule in a zombie movie out there. I myself love a good cardio workout, no this doesn't mean

I love to run. So many people think running on a treadmill or other machine is the only way to get cardio in. That simply isn't true. There is HIIT (high intensity interval training) Tabata, and many others. The idea is to get your heart going. Yes, cardio will help you burn fat, but it is also good for you. I make it a regular part of my fitness regimen and in the programming you see later it will be listed. Don't fear it! As I said before, cardio isn't the only way to get fit, with that being said I do still recommend it, it is good for you.

Chapter 5

Pushing to New Levels

I gotta tell ya, I love push-ups! I truly feel the push-up is the king of the chest workouts. So many muscles get to work all at once. You get to work your chest, shoulders, triceps, abs and many more in this one basic move. How cool is that? Through this section we will break down the best ways to progress your push, so everyone from beginner to

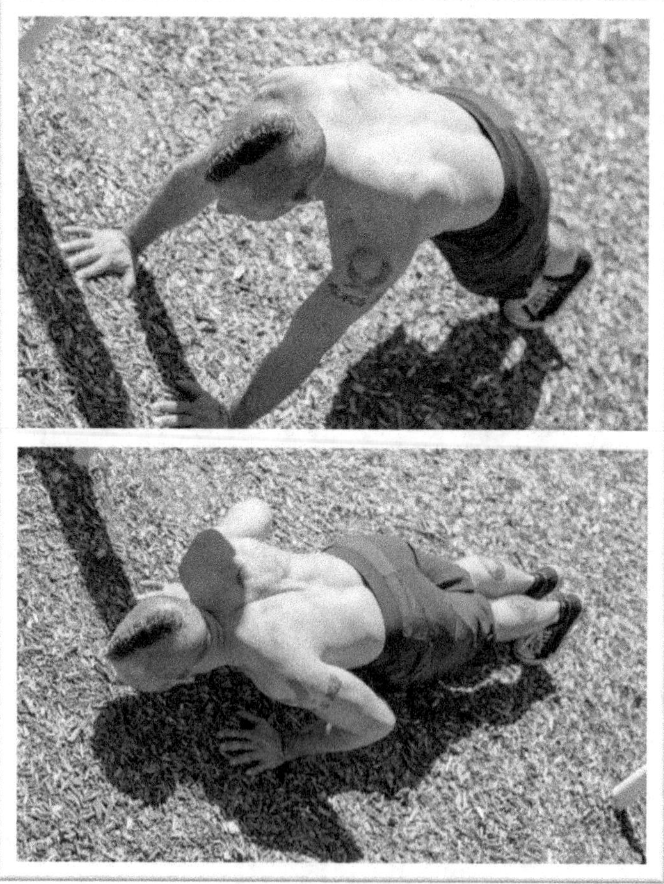

advanced can benefit from this key movement. You may think you can't do push-ups, but I'm going to show you that you can.

With the push-up, let's first talk about hand placement. One thing I see a lot of is hands placed too high. Sadly, this almost makes it a shoulder workout. So, before we even take this to the ground, let's look at hand placement. Your thumbs should be just about in line with your armpits. Look at the basic chest press. The bar goes across the chest, not the neck or shoulders. Now from here tuck your hips under and tighten your abs. Yes, you have abs. You just may not see them yet. To be honest this muscle engagement should be done with ever movement and every exercise. Let's take a moment and look at the push-up options for progression and regression.

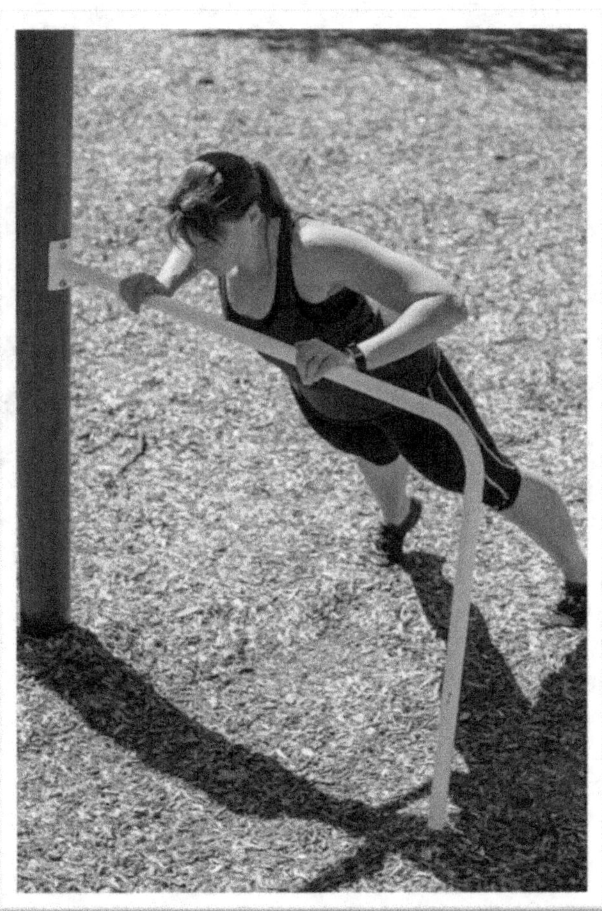

A lot of times I start people with incline push-ups. The increase in the angle takes some of the stress off the muscles while keeping your form intact. This can really be done anywhere! I have used a park bench, stairs, even the arm of my couch. Now, if the challenge is still too much, then you can also adjust your feet. Moving the feet apart will create more points of contact and potentially make the movement easier.

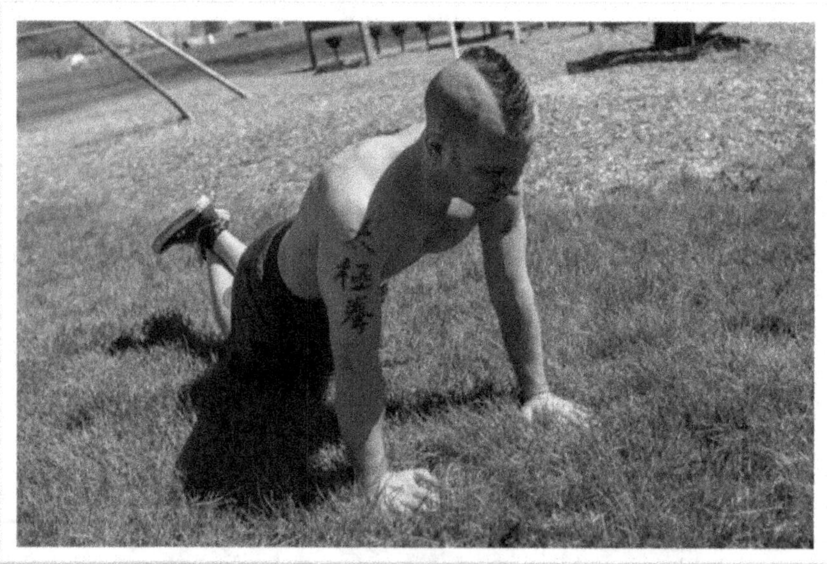

Another option when starting out is knee push-ups. Personally, I don't recommend these often, mostly due to the few issues I see. Just like all other push-ups you want to keep the core tight and many people hinge from the hips when it should be from the knee. If you choose to travel down this path, I would suggest starting out lying flat on the floor, then cross your ankles and bend the knees. From here push yourself up. Again, keep the muscles engaged.

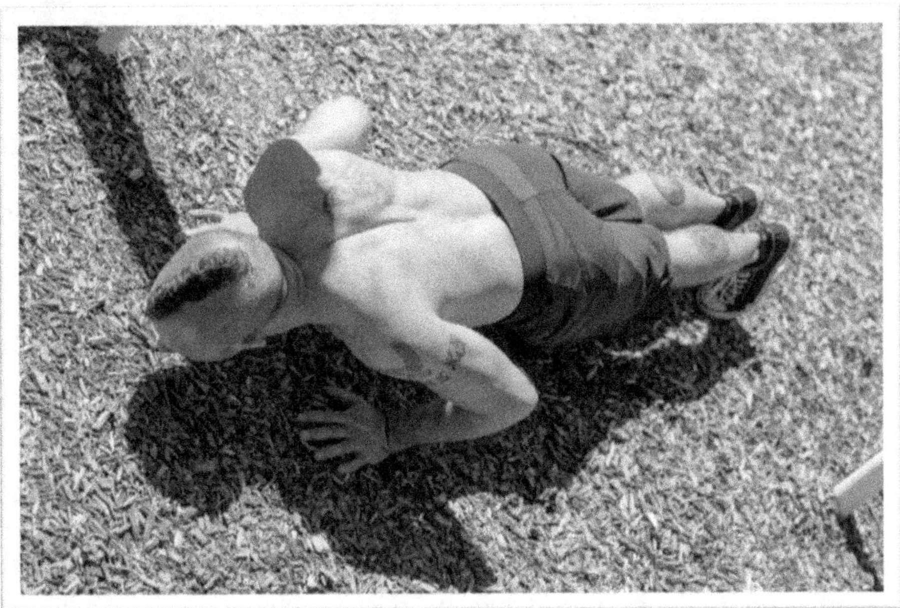

Once you feel you are ready for the next step, you can hit the classic push-up. I suggest if it is your first time doing a classic push-up, to try it with your feet apart. This should offer you a better base of support making the transition to the floor a little easier and you should be able to keep your form intact. To count a push-up as a rep, you need to at the very least get your arms to 90 degrees. Remember, there is nothing wrong with regression if it is necessary.

Time to level up! When those classic push-ups become too easy, there are a few things you can do. First off, you can do more reps or you can start playing with hand and foot position. Once your feet are together try moving your hands closer together. You will notice quickly, the closer your hands get the greater the challenge will be. Your 20 push-ups will quickly become 10. But, before you know it your hands will both be at the center of your chest. Another way to progress the classic push-up, is to do it with only one leg touching the ground. You can stack the feet, or just lift one. Either way, the fewer points of contact to the earth will make the challenge greater. I also suggest trying them on your knuckles for a greater challenge and the availability for a deeper range of motion.

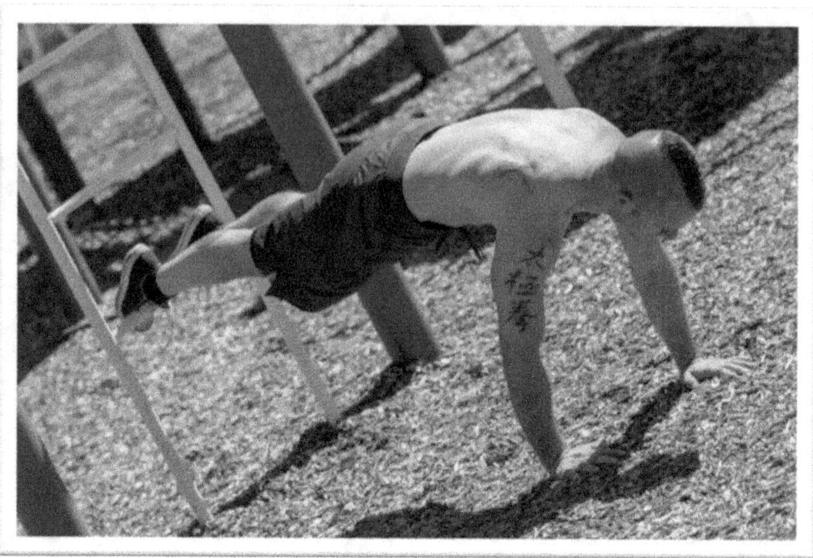

Another great progression is the decline push-up. Like some of the other progressions, you change the angle to change the difficulty. For this you can place your feet on a chair, bench or any other elevated surface and place your hands on the ground. As I keep saying, engage all your muscles and start your push-ups. You will notice the weight on your arms is now much greater.

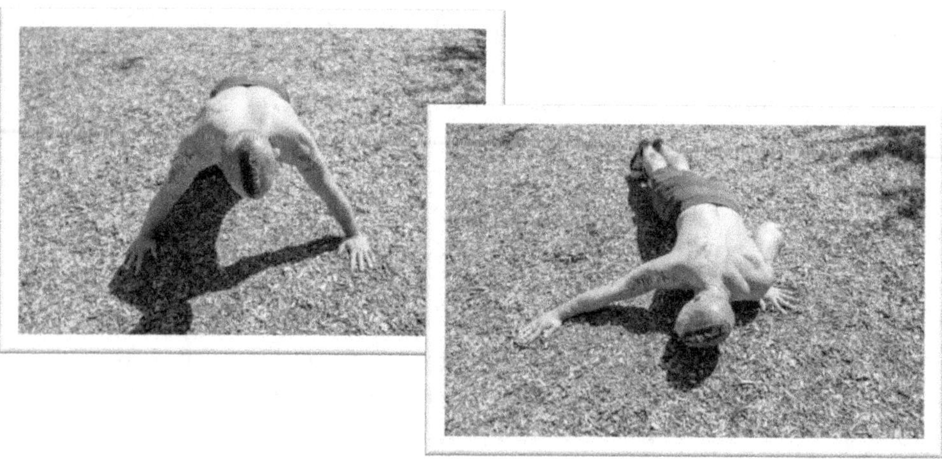

One of the push-ups I like to add into my workouts is the Archer Push-Up. This one can be a monster, so make sure you have good body control before you attack this one. The Archer Push-Up, you want to start with your arms a bit further apart, then lower yourself down on one side straightening the opposite arm, like an archer drawing a bow. Then push back up to center, and repeated on the other side.

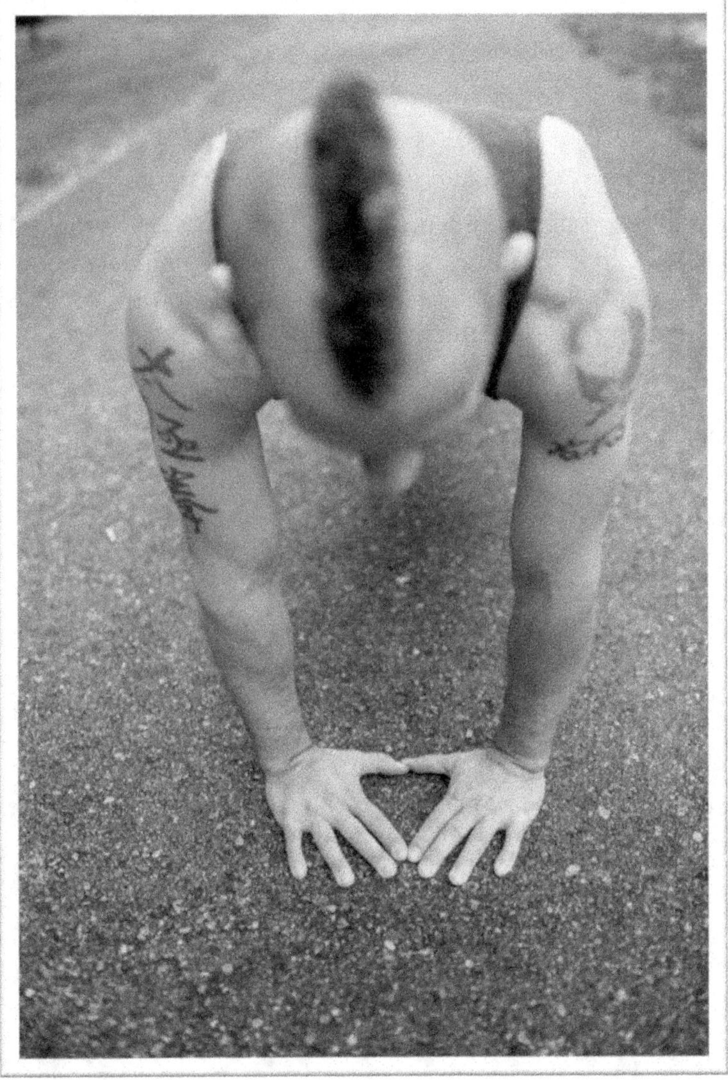

Diamond Push-Ups bring the hands together, thumb to thumb. Narrowing your hands like this will challenge your core stability. Start in your push-up position, and place both hands under the center of your chest, thumb to thumb and tip of index fingers together. As you lower yourself down, try to keep your elbows along your sides. It will be a challenge to keep them from flaring out. Then, push it back up.

The staggered hand push-up is a great progression towards the one arm push-up. Start in the classic push-up position, from here extend one arm out over head putting most of your weight on one arm. From here you do your push. After a few reps switch arm position. This will be a challenging push-up.

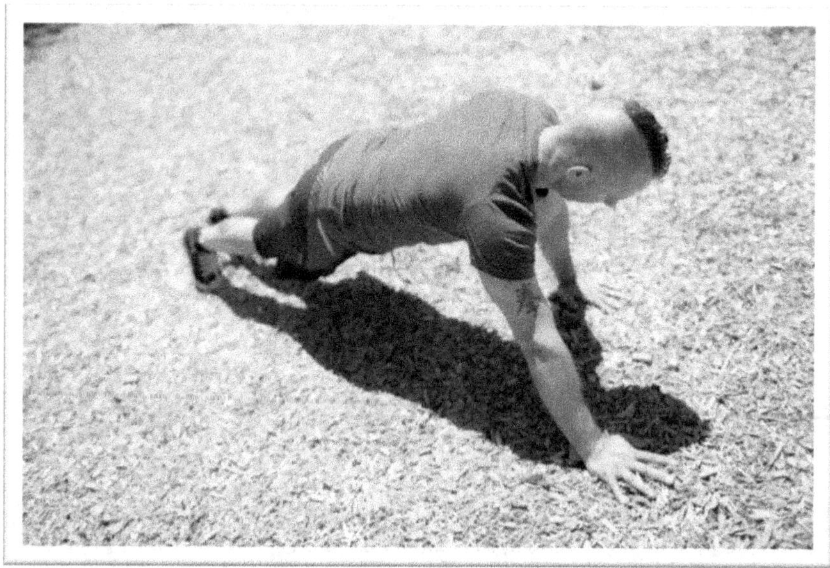

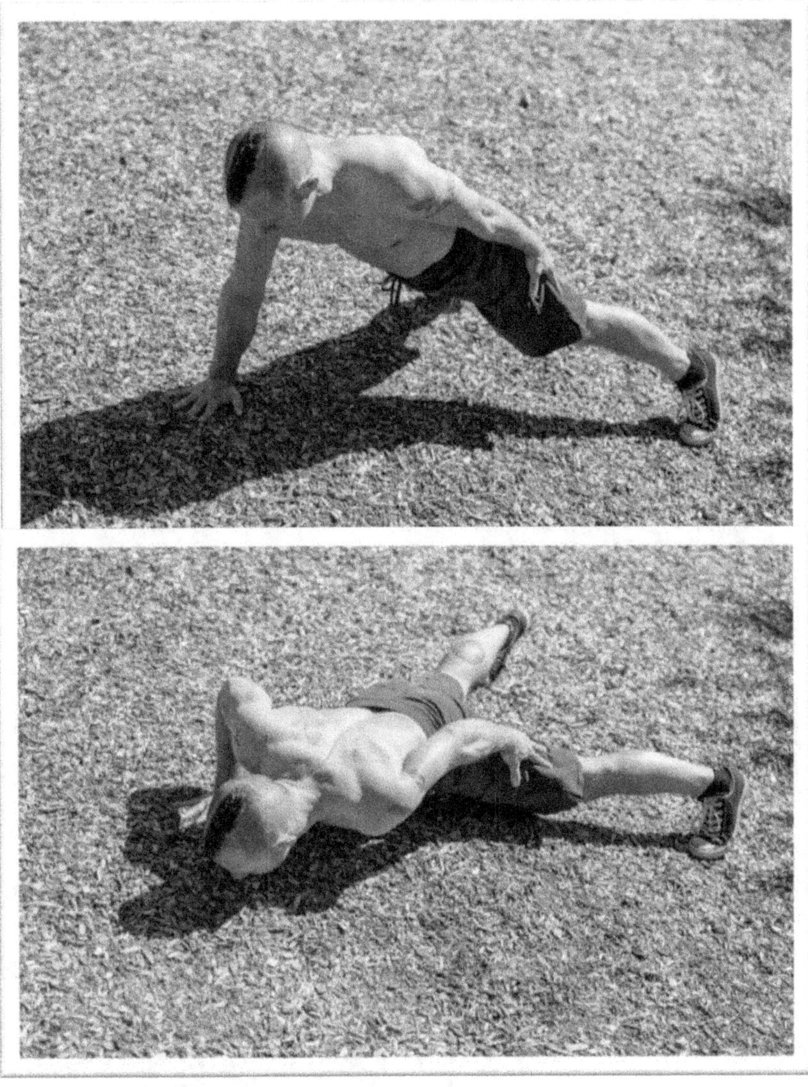

Here it is, the bad ass of the push-ups, the infamous one arm push-up! This journey will be rough, but it will be worth it in so many ways. Just like the regular push-ups, I suggest starting with your hands on an elevated surface, maybe even spread the feet apart. As you get stronger, you can go to lower and lower surfaces for your hands. Once on the ground, I suggest staggering your hands a bit, what this does is just offer better balance. Once you have the balance down, separate your feet and start pushing. The hardest part will be to keep your body from twisting. You need to control your body to get the best benefit from this. As you get stronger, you can once again ply with foot placement to boost the challenge.

One of my favorite trick push-ups is the hinge push-up. This starts as a normal push-up, then it evolves. As stated earlier, start in the push-up position and lower yourself down. Once at the bottom, roll down to tap your elbows in the floor. Then, roll back up and push back up.

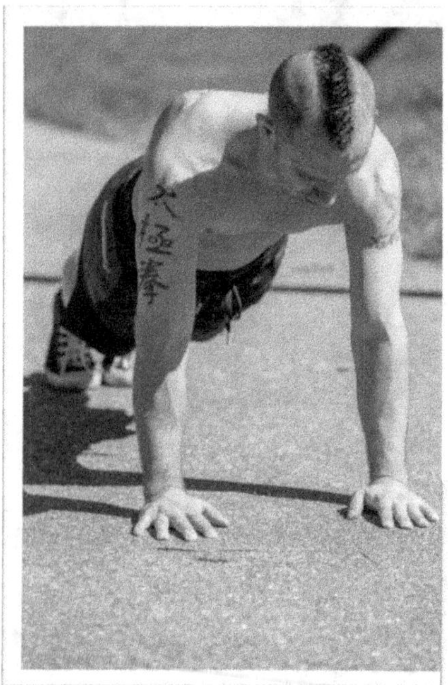

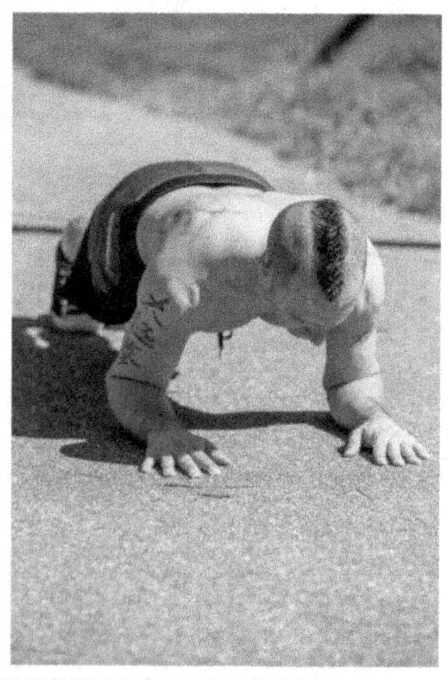

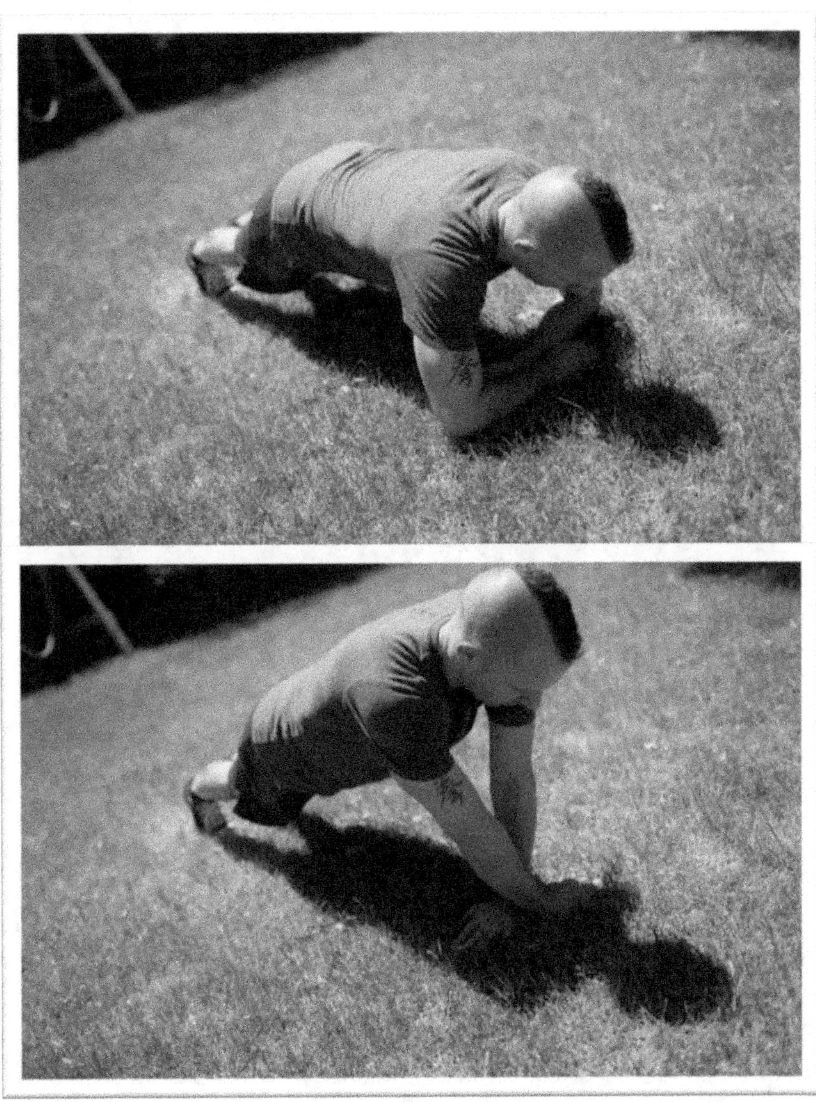

Cross Hand Push-Ups are a challenge similar to the hinge push-ups. Cross your hands wrist to wrist, as you get stronger you can go as far as wrist to elbow. Once here lower yourself down until your elbows touch the floor. I would suggest having padding for your elbows when first trying this. Once at the bottom push yourself back up. Remember to switch what hand is in front to keep it even.

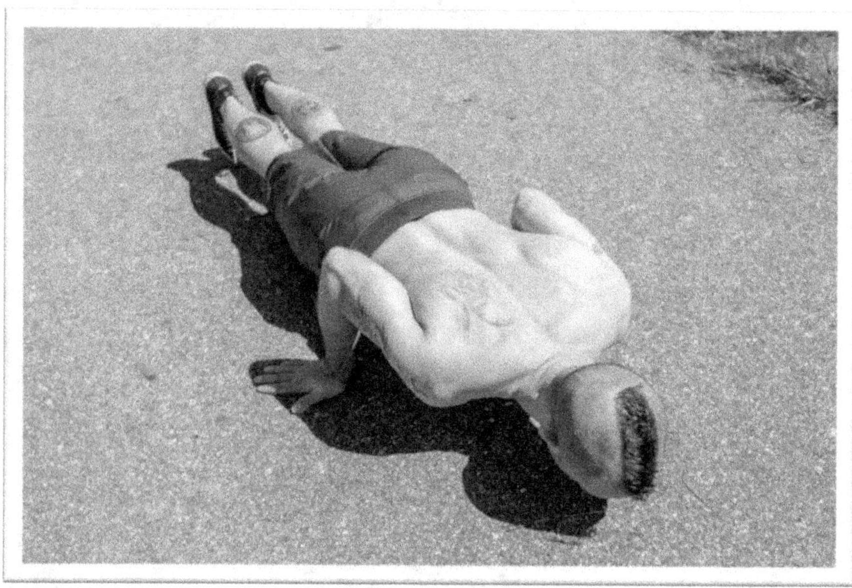

Planche Push-Ups, also nicknamed faceplants, are a unique monster. These start with the hands closer to the waist and turned backwards. You should be able to now understand why they can be called faceplants! From this position, you lower down and back up.

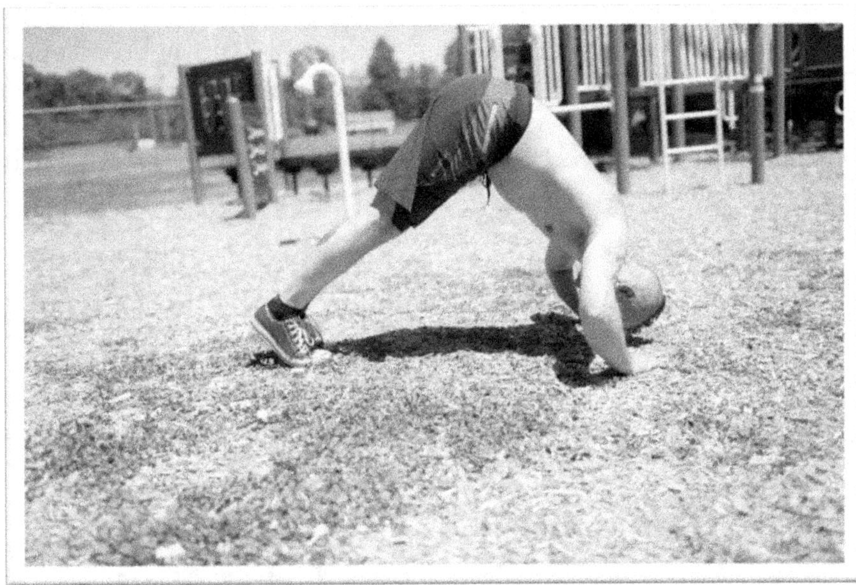

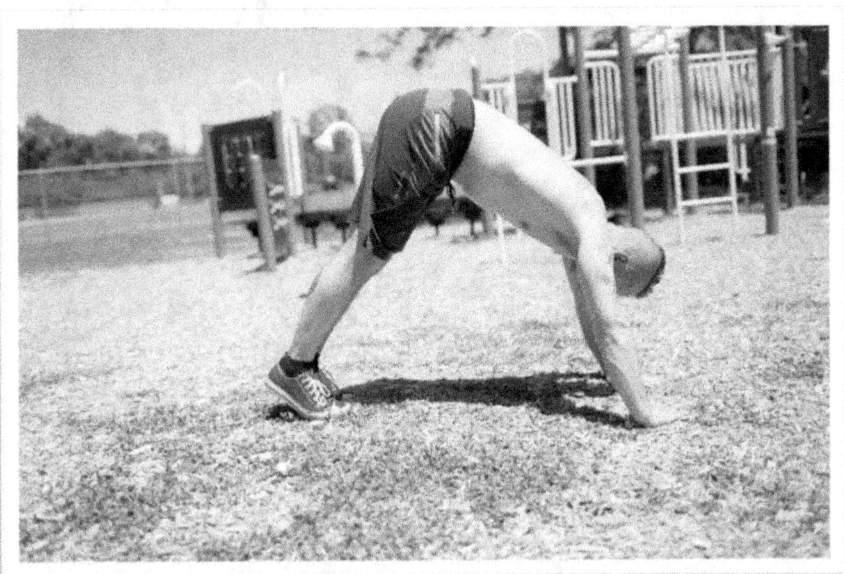

Pike Press Push-Ups are great for building the strength in your shoulders. To start walk your feet close to your hands and hike your butt up in the air, at this point it is ok to be up on your toes. Once in this position lower your head down between your hands and push back up.

Elevated Pike Press Push-ups are the next step up, almost literally. The body position is about the same except your feet will be on an elevated surface such as a chair or a bench. The stress on your shoulders will for sure be higher. Once in position lower yourself down between your hands and push back up.

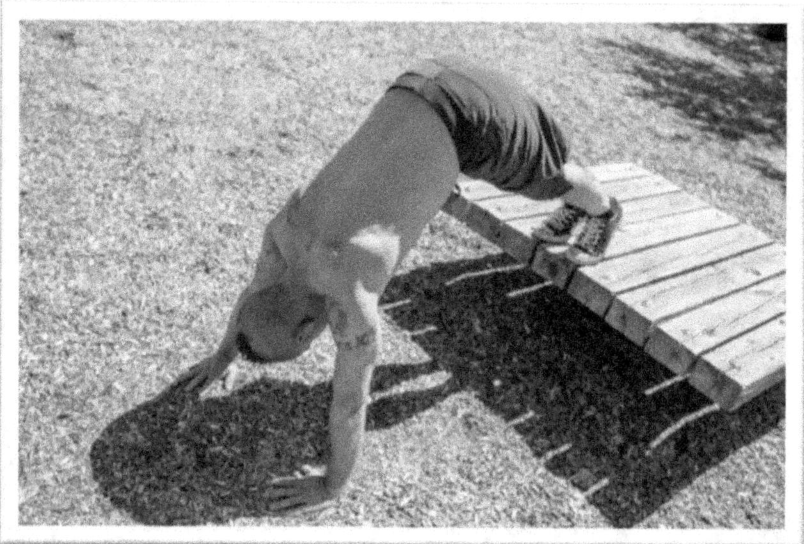

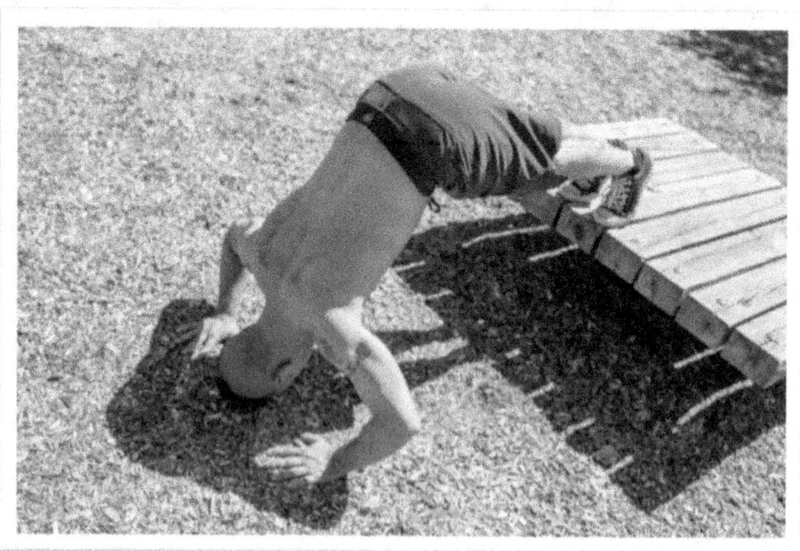

Hand Stand Push-ups make it feel like you are holding the entire world up with your hands. I highly, highly suggest using the wall to do

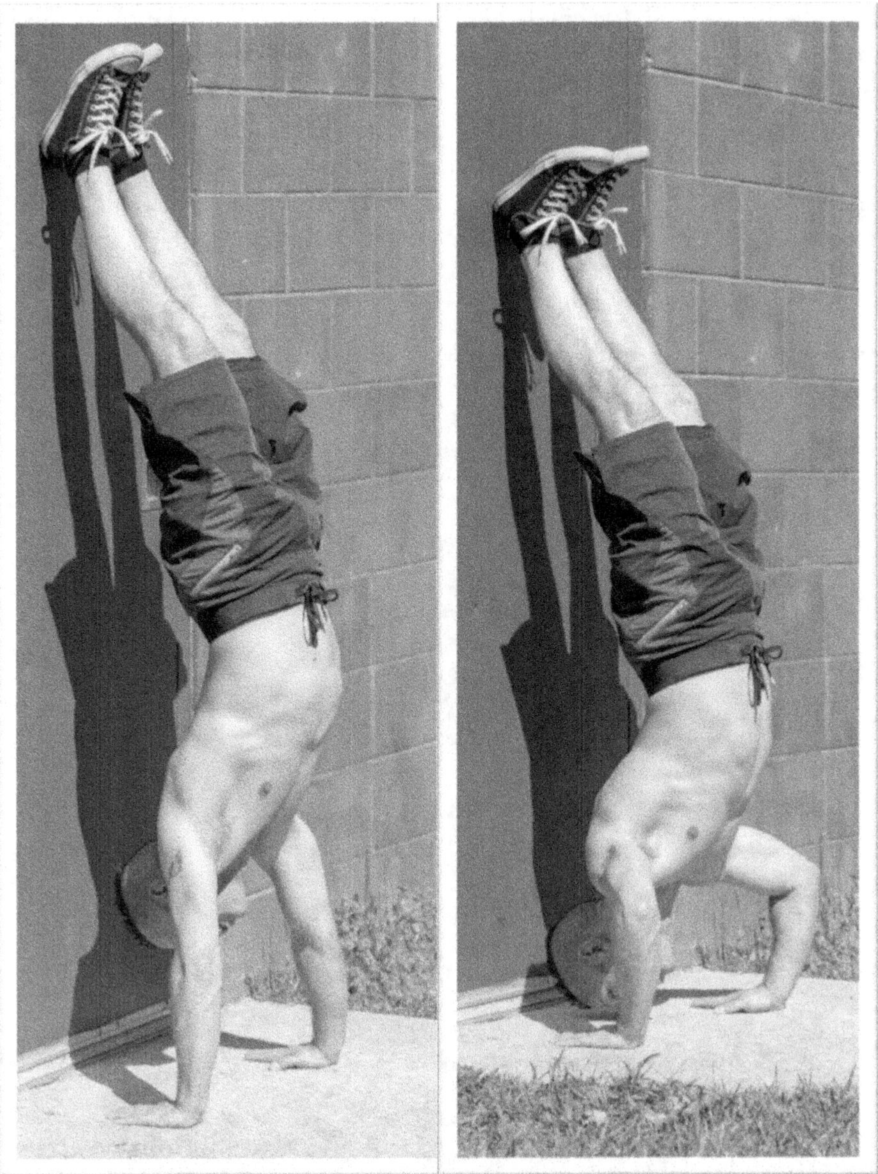

this. Also, be sure to warm up those wrists. To start, get yourself into your hand stand, from here lower yourself down between your hands and push yourself back up.

Bench Dips are your next push, and is great for beginners, but it can really be beneficial for all levels. To get started find an elevated surface, such as a bench, and place your hands on the bench behind your back. From here bend your knees, and lower yourself down bending from the elbows and shoulders keeping your torso straight, then push back up. Try not to shrug your shoulders on dips. Other variations would be doing the bench dips with the legs straight or straight legs on an elevated surface to increase the difficulty on the arms.

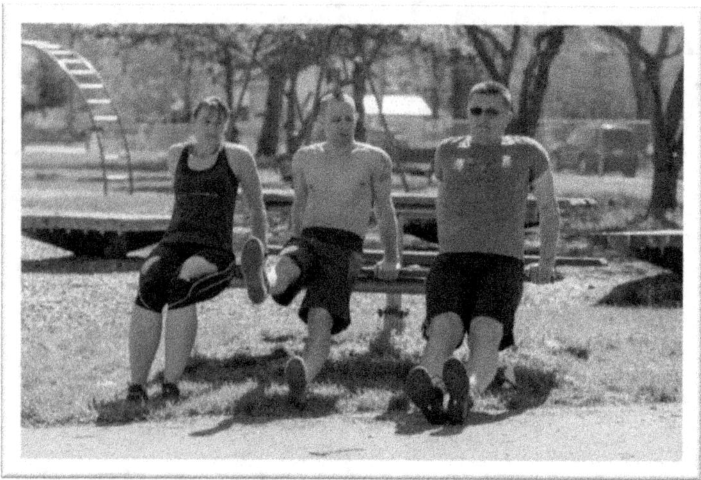

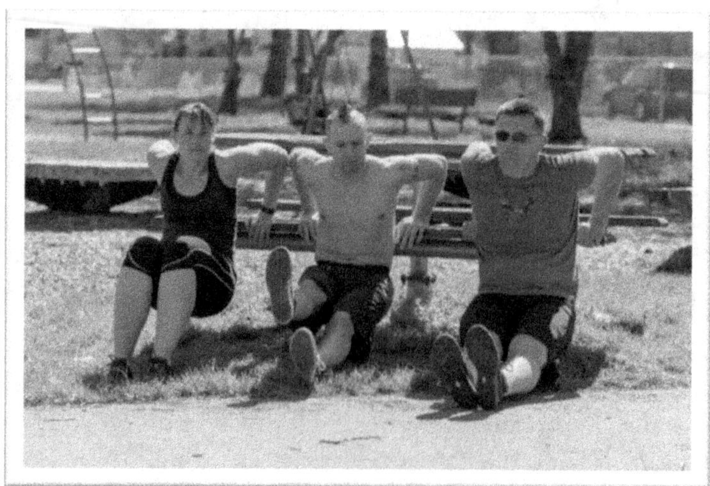

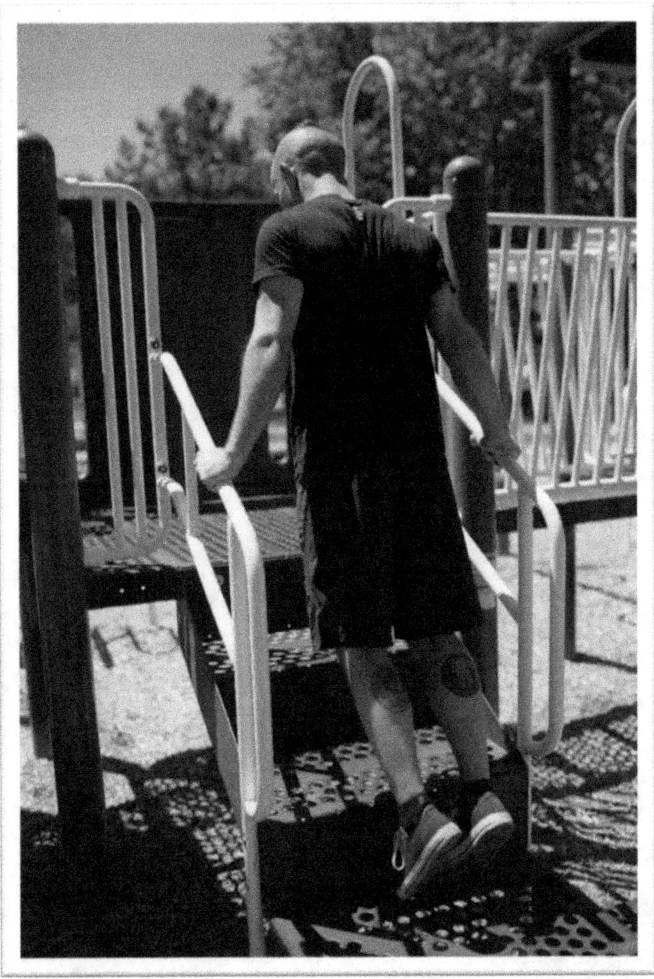

Parallel Bar Dips put you back on the bar. It's just what it sounds like, dips on parallel bars. First up, find a set of bars about shoulder width apart, then lift yourself up off the ground. As you lower yourself down between the bars, bend from the elbows and shoulders, but try not to shrug. Focus on getting the elbows to point behind you and not flaring out. You may see people at the gym bending their legs as they do this, but you are training to be a super hero. Keep the legs straight and hollow the body. But, if by chance it is too challenging, bending the knees will make it a little easier. Also, if you lean slightly forward it will move stress a bit more to the chest, but if you can keep vertical, you will rock the triceps.

Straight Bar Dips are done with a single bar in front of you. With both hands on the bar in front of you, bend at the hips a bit to fold over the bar and lower yourself down pointing the elbows behind you. As you get closer to the bottom you may also have to move the legs forward too. Then push yourself back up. This will be challenging now that there is balance involved.

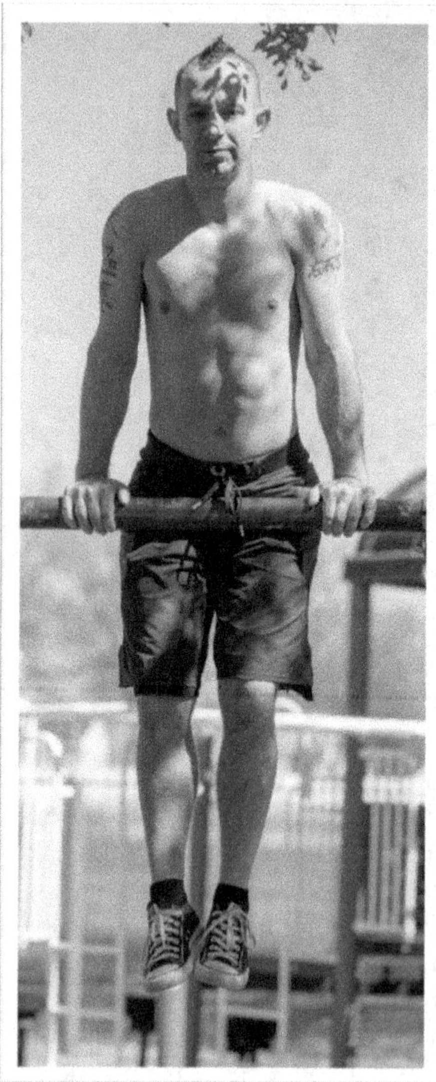
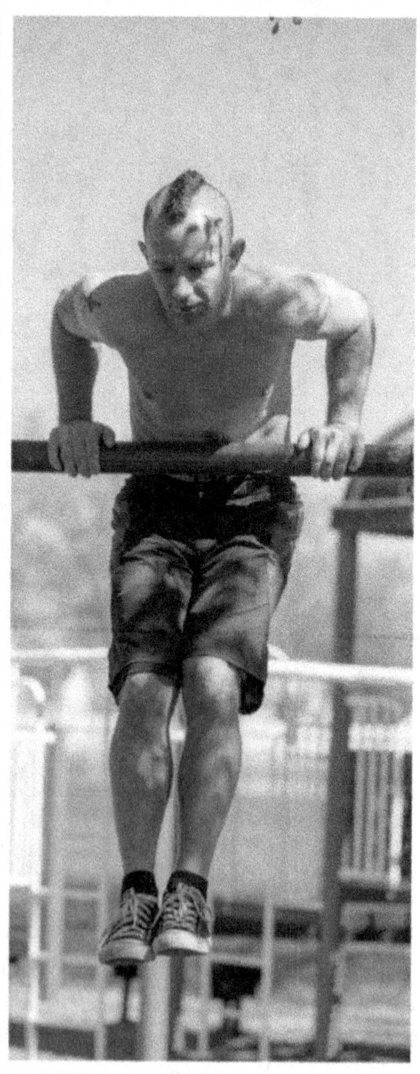

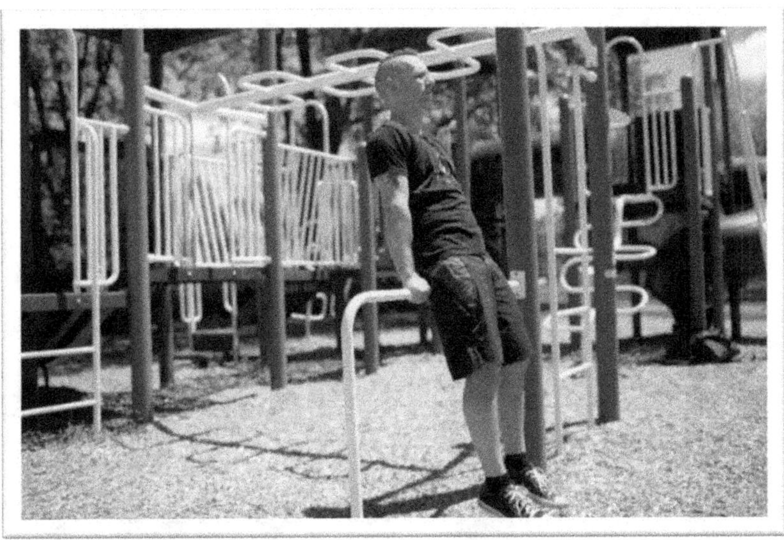

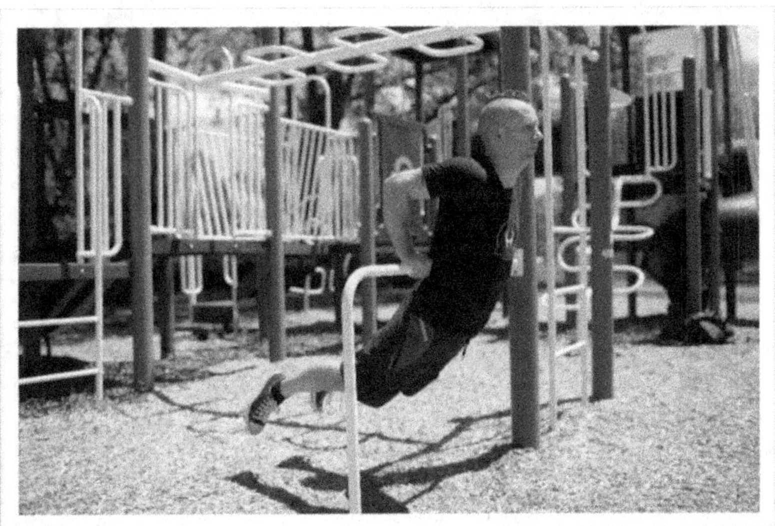

Korean Dips are one of the hardest dips to perform, in my opinion. I give you this warning: make sure you are good with the prior dip movements and your shoulders are ready for this because your body will be suspended on a bar behind your back. Hands gripping the bar behind your back, tighten your abs and engage the entire core. As you lower yourself down you will slowly you will slightly swing under the bar, then push back up. As I said, this will be a great challenge and should be done carefully.

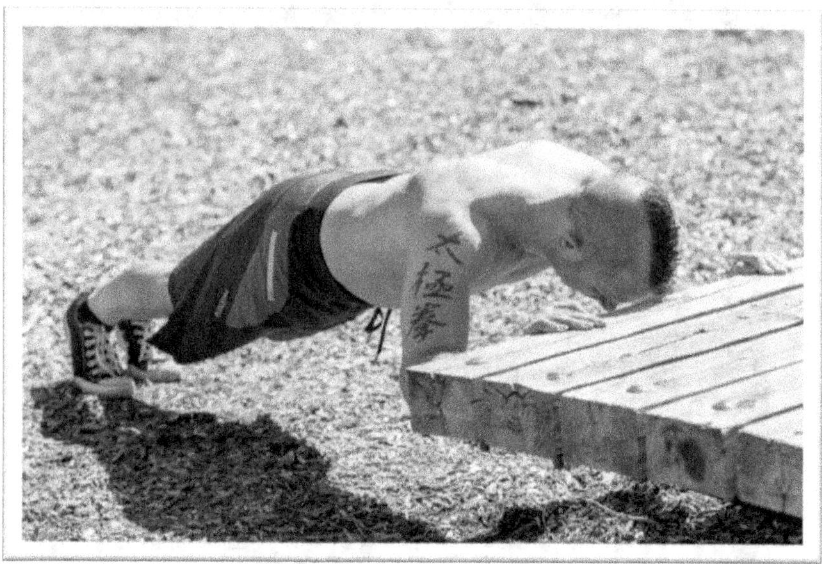

Reverse Skull Crushers... I feel the name alone is epic. This one can be done on a bar or bench that is low to the ground. Place your hands on the bench or bar as if you are doing an elevated plank. From here bend the elbows lowering your head towards the bar or bench then push it back up.

Chapter 6
Pull-ups

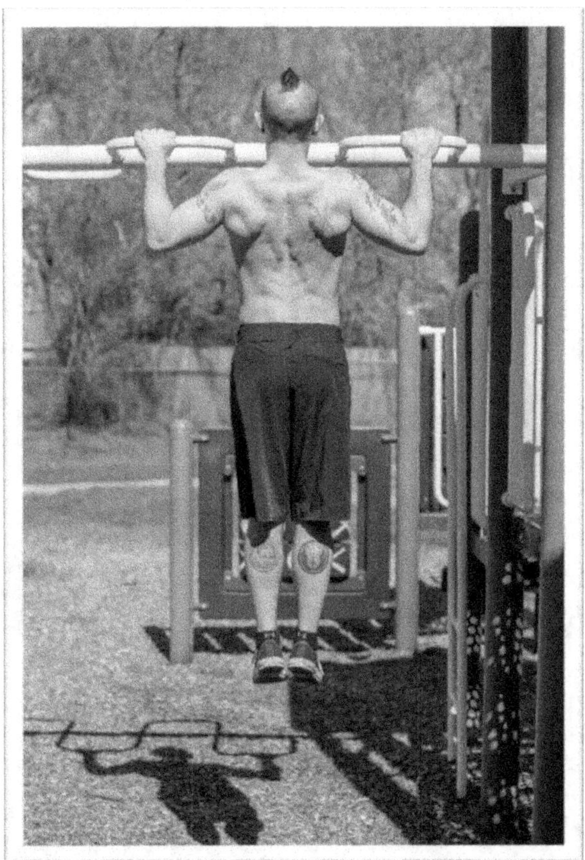

Pull-ups may be one of the hardest exercises out there. Not everyone can do them, and a lot of people that claim to do them don't do them correctly. Like the push-up, the pull-up engages a lot of muscles all at once such as a lot of the back, shoulder and biceps, and if you engage it properly you can also get your abs. The pull-up can also be modified to increase or decrease the difficulty, as well as focus the tension a little differently. Just like the push-ups, the entire body should be engaged. After all, why only work a small amount of muscles when you can work many? So, for the pull-up start with arms fully extended hanging from the bar, from here you pull yourself all the way up until the chin clears the bar then lower yourself all the way down until arms are extended fully. That, my friends, is a full rep. One thing I have done in the past when training for my Pull-Ups, was to use resistance bands or Pull-Up assist bands. They ease up the weight while still giving you that Pull-Up motion. If you go this route, try to get yourself off of them as soon as you can.

Like I said before, not everyone is ready for pull-ups. One good way to work towards them is with Bodyweight Rows or Aussie pull-ups. With this angle is key. Want more difficulty? Go further under the bar. With this back workout, I have used everything from a kitchen table, to a park bench. This one has a lot of room to play around. You can bend your legs to make the exercise easier or straighten them out to up your challenge. But, like the pull-up, range of motion is everything. For a beginner, it's not a bad idea to choose a bar about chest height, and as your strength score increases, you can go lower to the ground. It's also not a bad idea to play with hand grip, narrow, wide and reverse grip are all acceptable. Start with arms at full extension, and pull your chest towards the bar pulling your shoulder blades

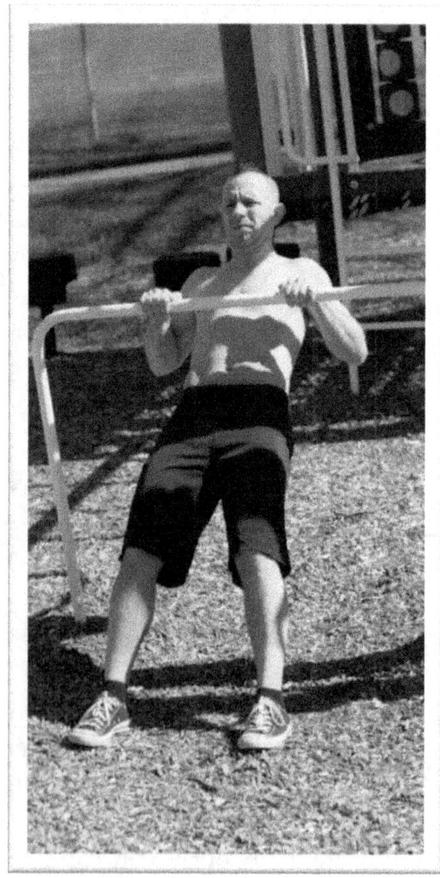

together. From here lower yourself back down until your arms are at full extension.

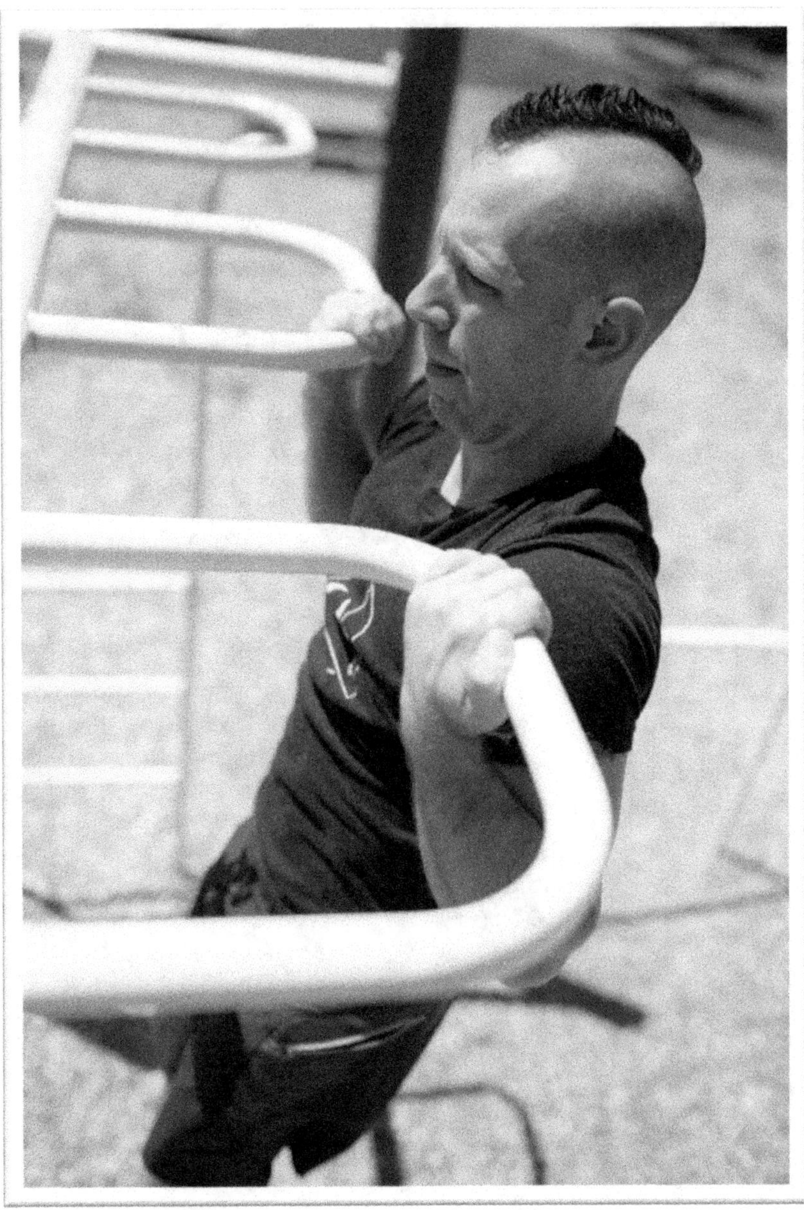

The Chin-Up is not much different than the pull-up; the main difference is your hands are reversed. With this change you will get a little extra pull from the biceps. Just like the pull-up, you want to start from a full hang, tighten your abs and pull your chin up over the bar then back down to full extension.

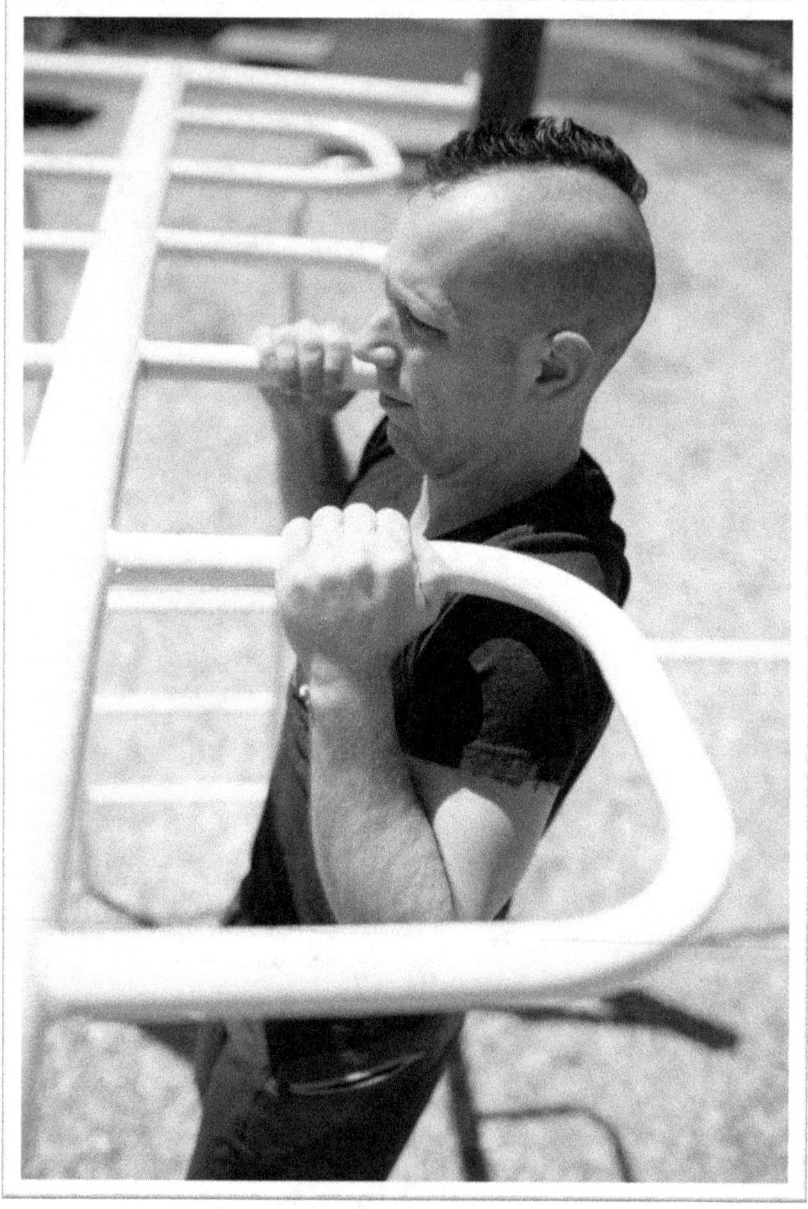

Neutral Pull-ups use bars that are parallel to each other and palms facing. Like the chin-up, this will have more aid from your biceps. For some this may be a little easier and more comfortable. Regardless of how well you can knock out standard pull-ups, you should try to throw these in from time to time.

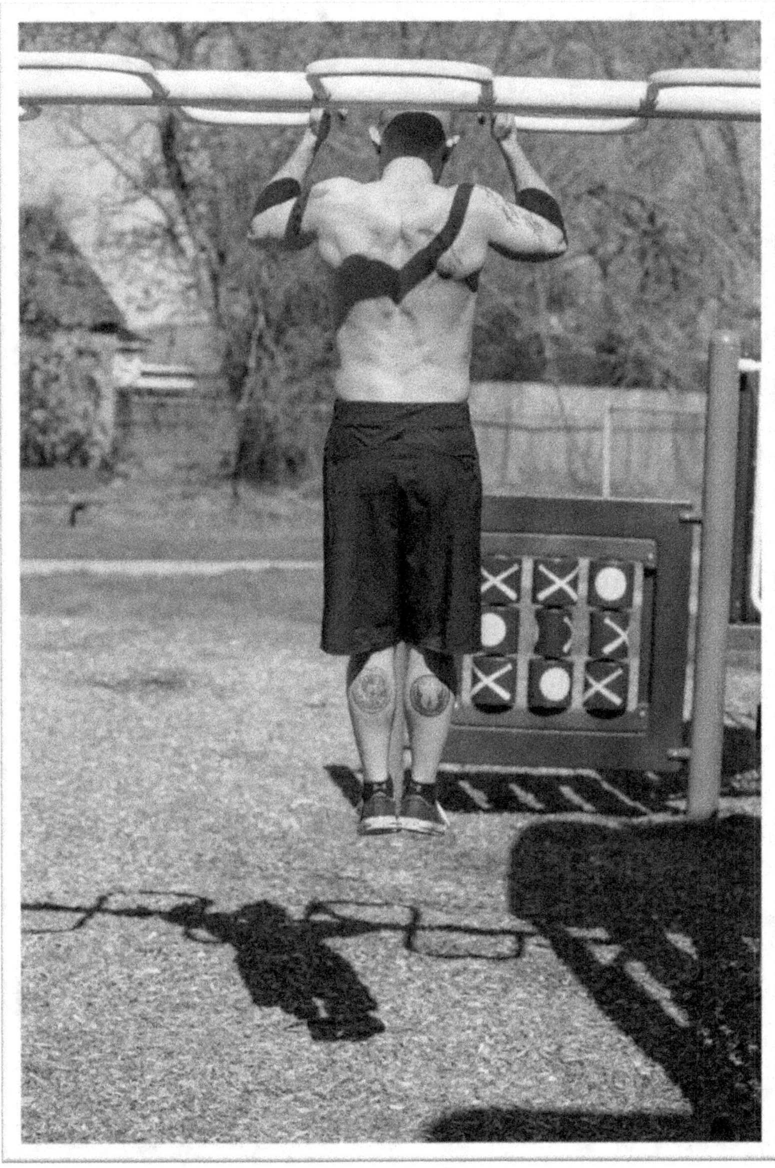

The behind the neck pull-up isn't always recommended unless you have great range or motion in your shoulders. I would also stay clear of it is you have standing neck issues. That being said, if you decide to give it a go, it is accomplished just like the classic pull-up but the bar goes behind the head instead of under the chin.

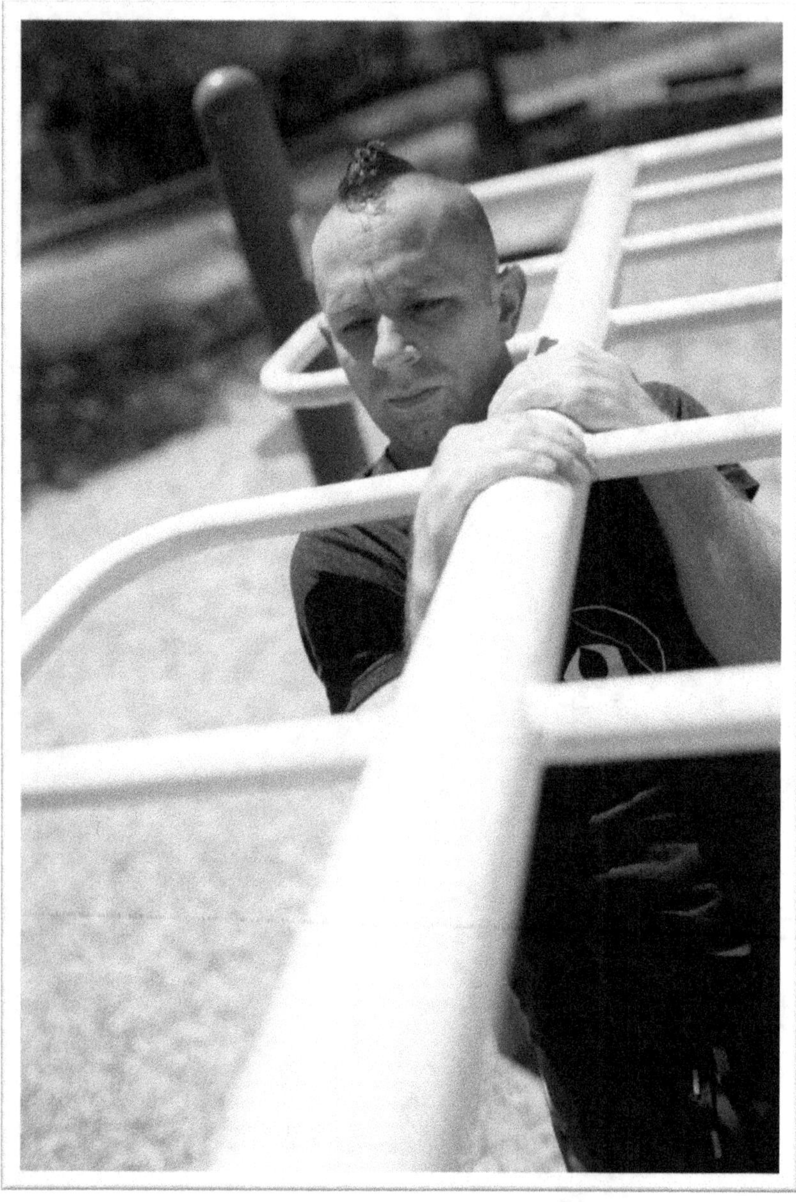

Commando Pull-ups have a grip similar to the neutral grip pull-up, but you use a single bar with your hands end on end. Since your body will be directly under the bar, pull the bar shoulder to shoulder. I would also suggest switching hand positions each set. You must keep it even, after all.

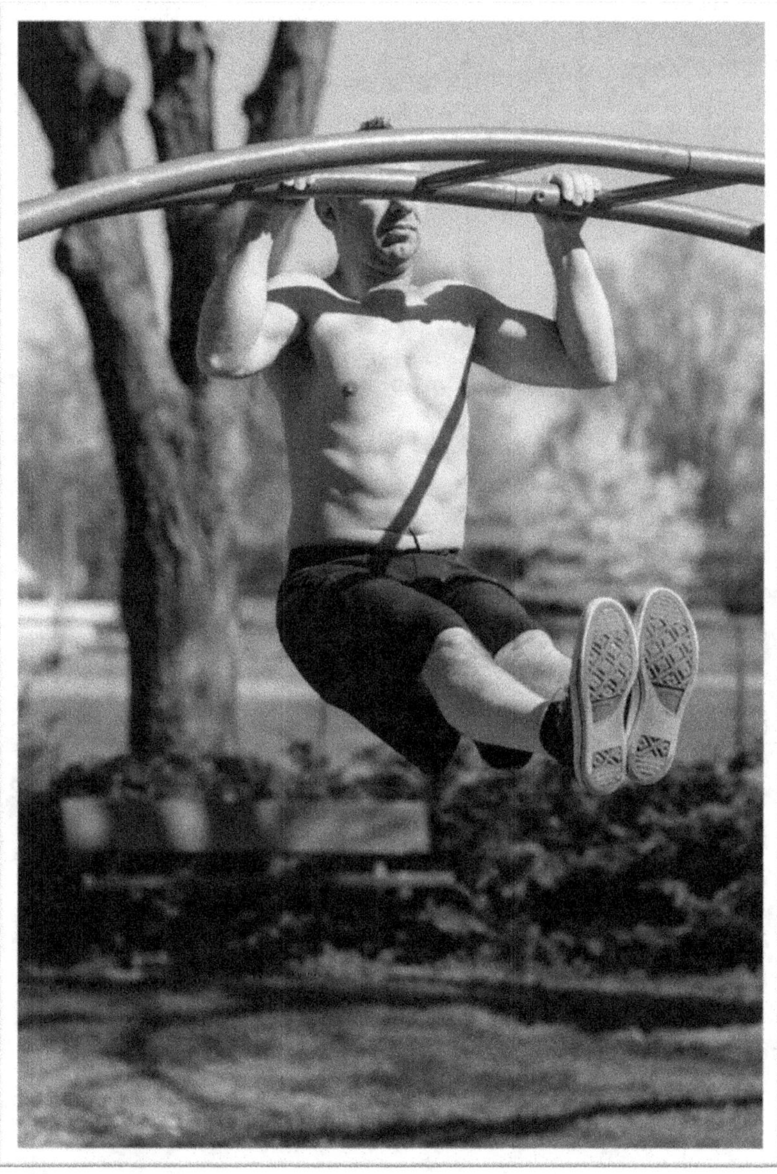

L-Sit Pull-Ups are a great way to change the game with the classic pull-up movement. When you bring your legs up to a 90 degree angle, you hit your abs, hip flexors and quads. This will also severely change the balance of the move. This move could easily be added to the Chin-ups, Commando and Neutral Grip. When ready, try to experiment a little.

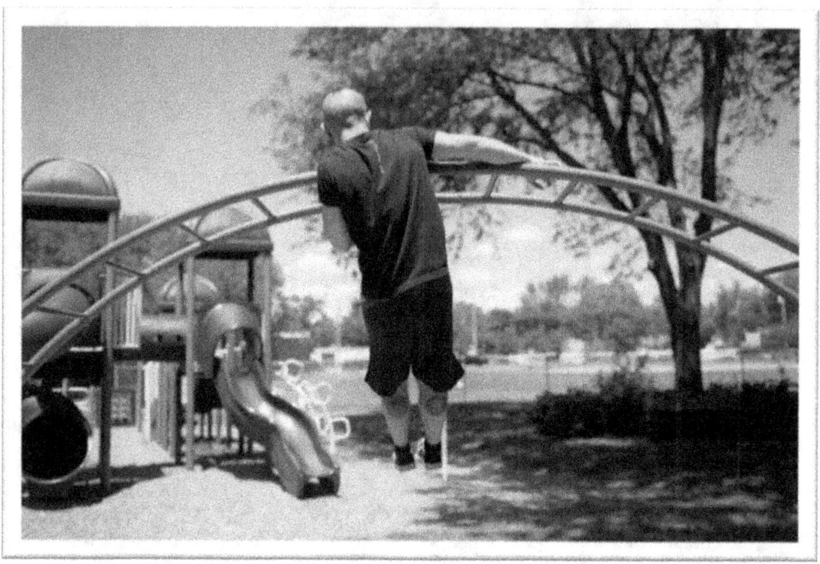

Archer pull-ups, like the push-up, you use one arm for the primary movement while the second arm stabilizes. So, while hanging on the bar, pull yourself up to one side and try to straighten the other arm. Now at first the empty arm may not go straight, but that's ok. It will come in time. Then you want to repeat it on the other side.

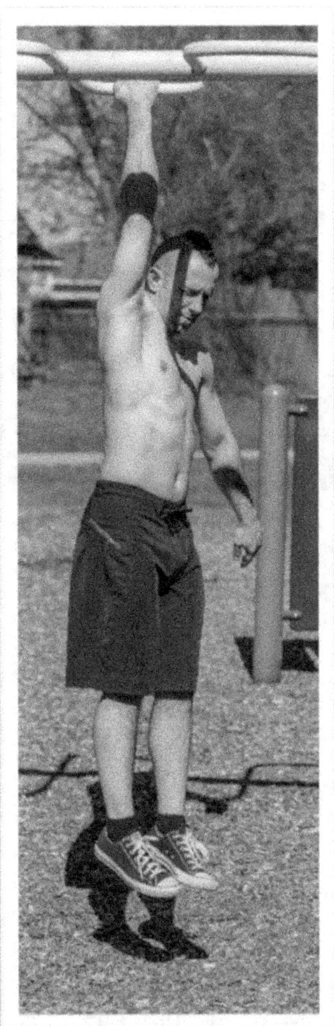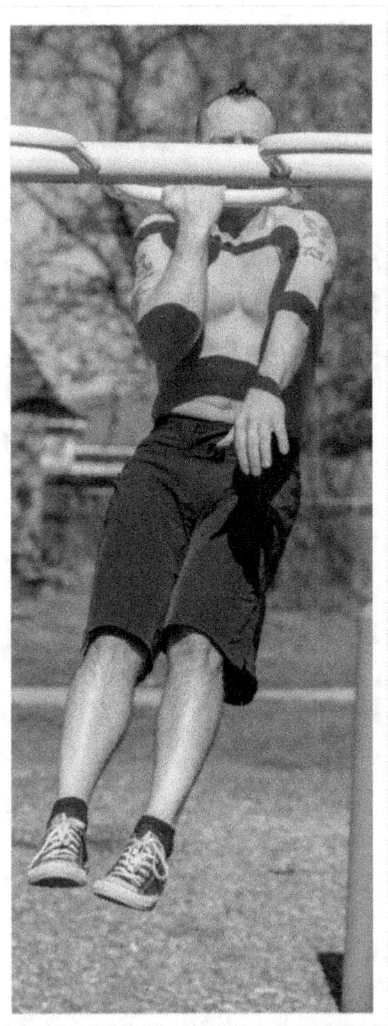

One arm pull-ups are a monster, and will take a lot of training to defeat! But there are steps to get you there. First off, you have to be able to nail a lot of pull-ups. Then, you have to work that grip with just hanging from the bar with one arm. Yeah, it doesn't seem like much, but try it. From there, pull yourself up to the top, and do a one arm flex hang. Once you can hold those for a while, start getting negative. What that means is, pull yourself up and lower yourself down slow. You could also do a supported one arm pull. This can be done by supporting your wrist with your other arm.

Chapter 7
Planks

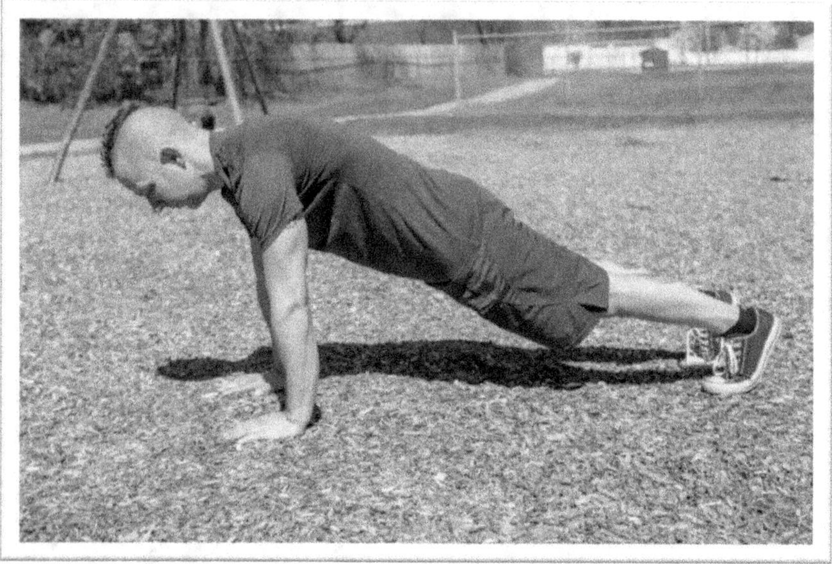

Everyone has seen a plank, but they are not just a core exercise. They are an entire body workout if done correctly. Just like so many other calisthenics moves, they can be progressed and regressed. Let's start this mission with the basics, the High Plank (aka the Push-Up Plank). The hands and feet should be on the floor, with the hands under the shoulders. Once at the top of this tuck your hips and engage your abs. Hold this position as long as you can. Plank hold variations will be important in all of this because some of the trickier moves use them to stabilize the body.

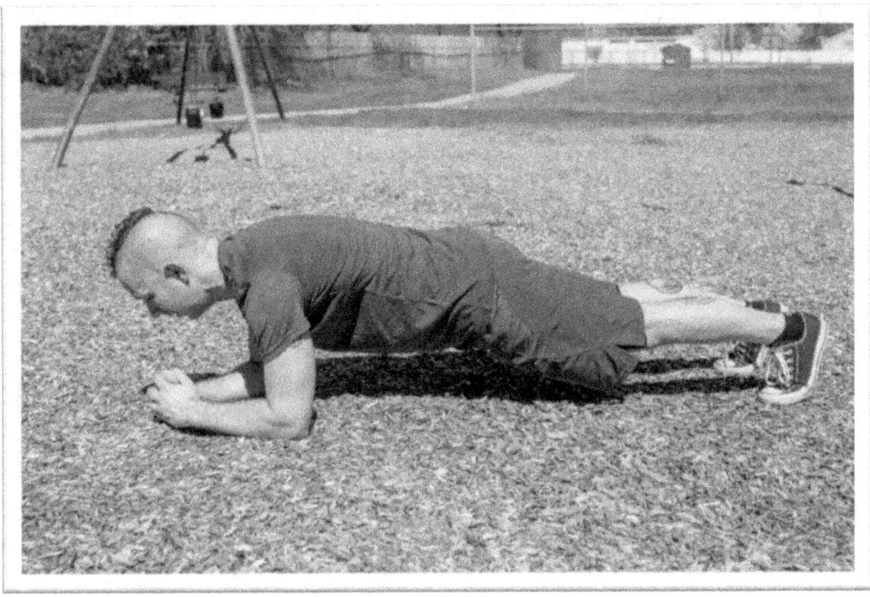

Low planks are one of my favorites to train. The main difference between the high plank and the low plank is, the low plank is on the elbows changing the angle. Make sure to keep those hips tucked and the elbows directly under the shoulders.

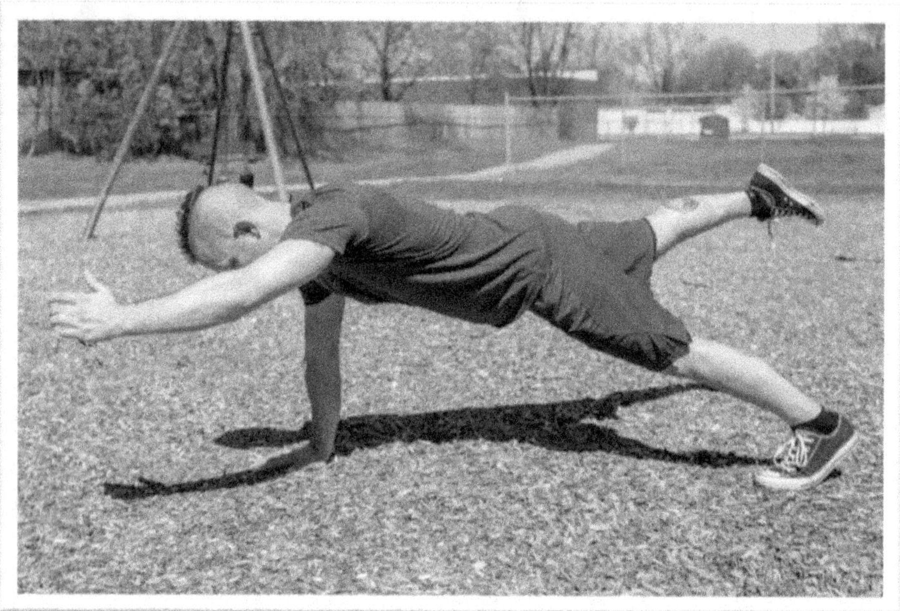

Just like everything else, you can progress this further. The Balanced Plank is a good step up. There are a few ways to progress this, you can start with taking one arm off the ground or one leg. It is important that you reduce the twist in the body as much as possible. Once you are ready, take one hand and one foot off the ground. Finding the balance on that will be a great challenge.

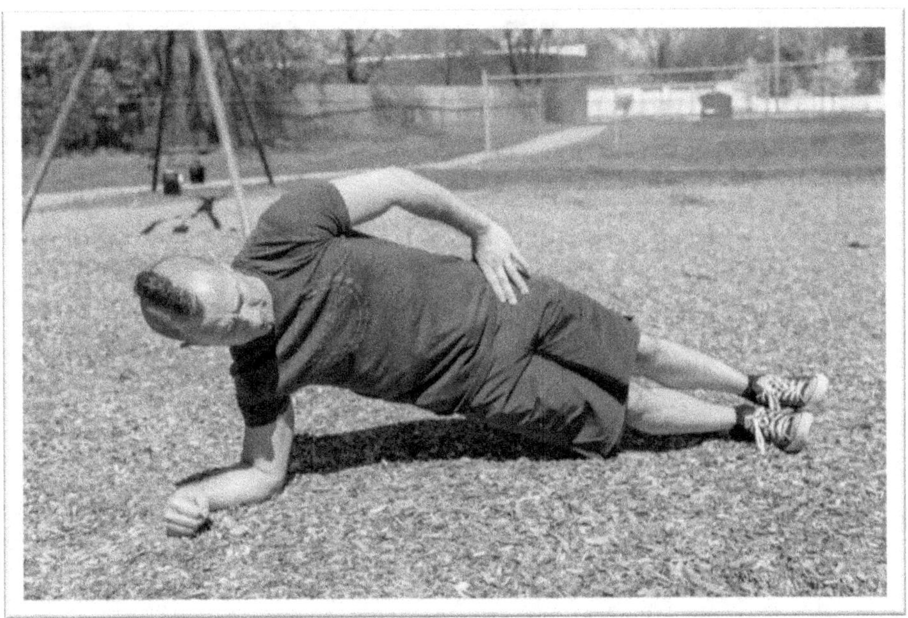

Side planks are great for building up that rib meat. The form for this is crucial. You need to keep your elbow directly under your shoulder and keep the hip up off the ground. Keeping your weight on your one elbow and your foot, try to hold this on both sides. One way to boost the challenge on these is to slightly elevate your feet.

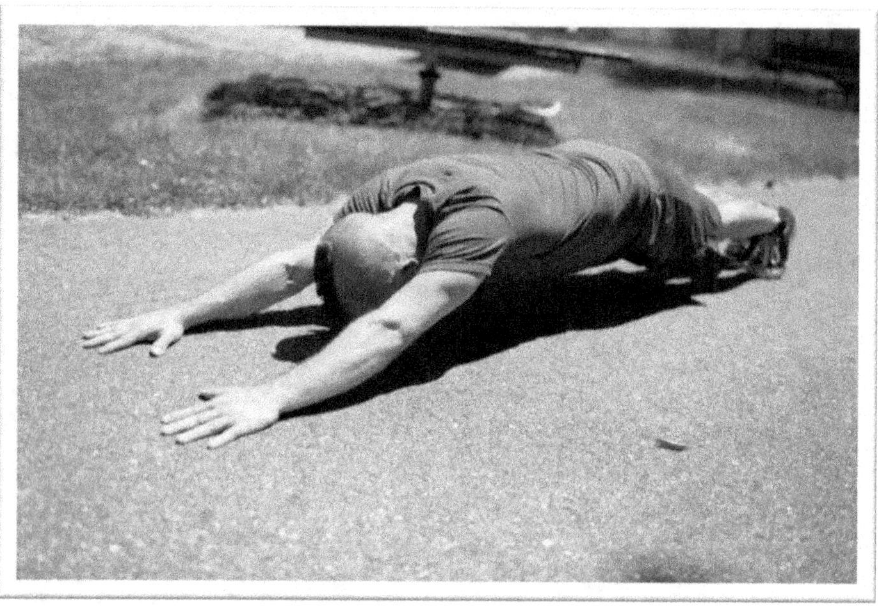

Superman Planks are rough, but are a great way to amp up that super hero core workout. To start, get yourself into a low plank, make sure your core is tight. Once here, you need to extend your arms out straight and hold yourself up with your hands and toes. This may put a lot of stress on the shoulders, so you may need to work up to it. Get that steel core!

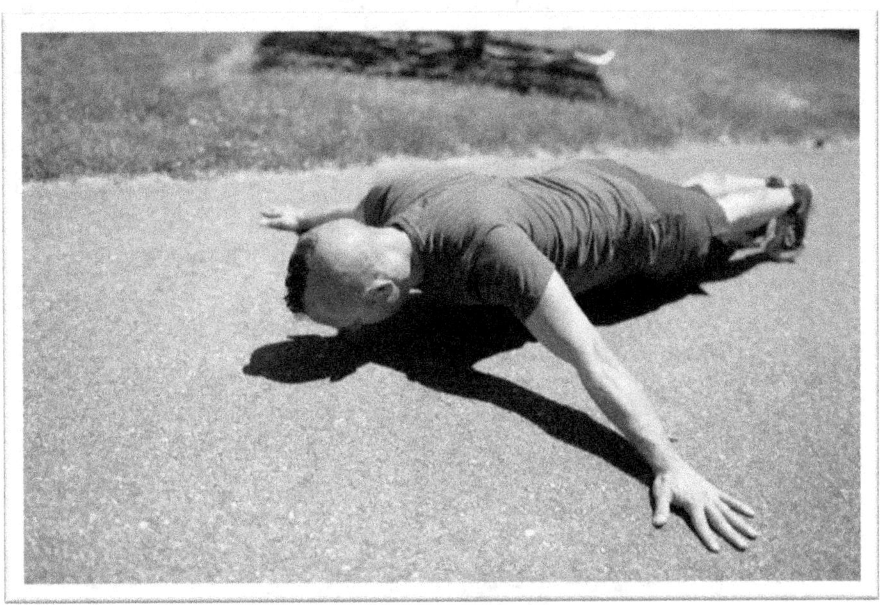

Airplane Planks require a lot of shoulder, arm and core strength. Starting in a low plank, tighten your core and hollow it out. From here Extend your arms out to the side like an airplane and hold yourself up on your palms and toes.

Chapter 8
You Can Skip With the Legs, But Don't Skip the Legs

Let's start it off with Squats. These may be the most important movement for your legs. It hits the entire leg if done right. But let's talk about them a little first, because I hear complaints about them a lot. Complaints like, "they hurt my knees" or "that movement is unnatural". First off, if they are causing you knee pain, then they can be modified, but odds are it is not your knees, it is the muscle above those knees, but as always listen to your body. Now as far as this being "unnatural", that is far from true. Riddle me this, what does a child do to pick something up off the ground? That's right! They squat! And they do it without being taught. Seems like they may be natural after all.

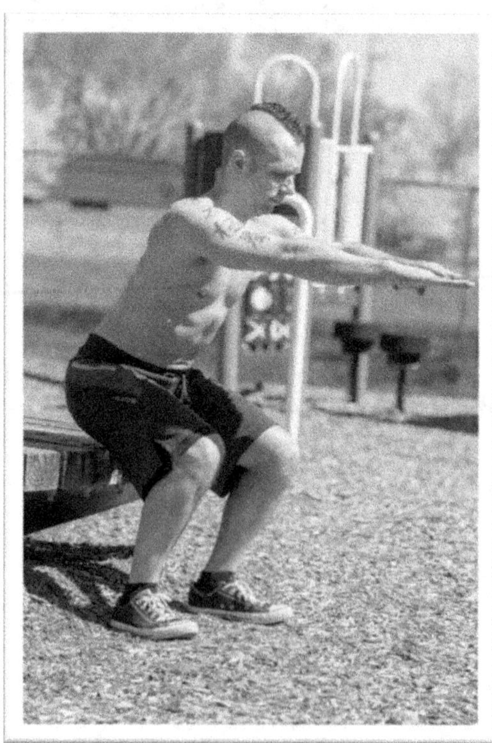

Before we look at those deep squats, let's look at how to modify them. One of the best starting points is the seated squat. This gives you the benefits of the squat, but the security of a chair to keep you from falling over. As you get stronger and more stable, the surface your butt hits can get lower. You could also use a pole to help yourself down and up for extra balance.

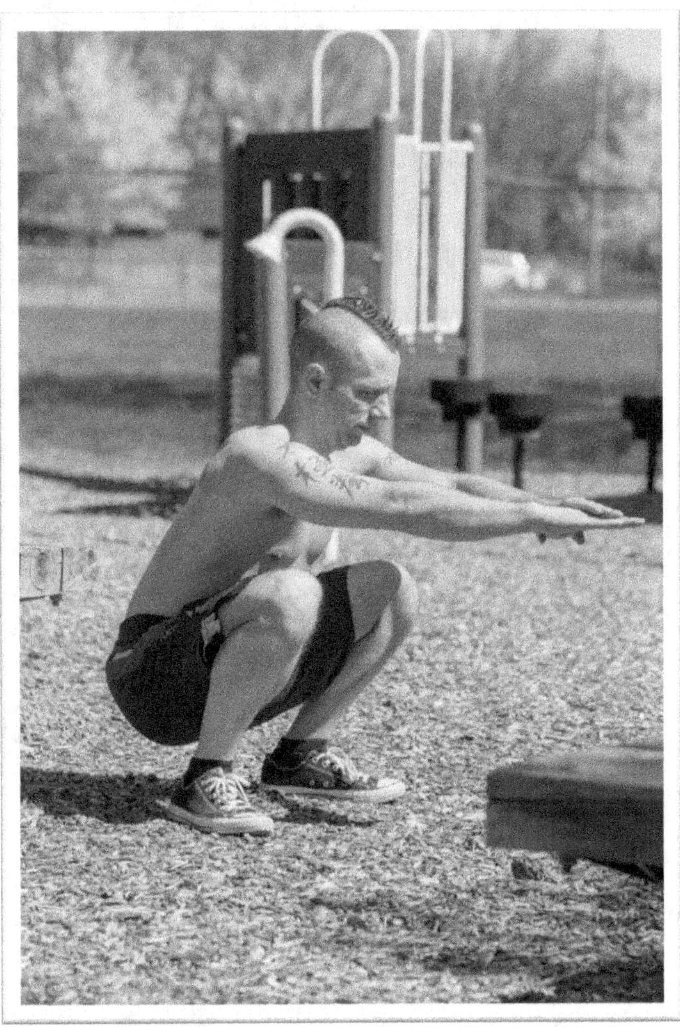

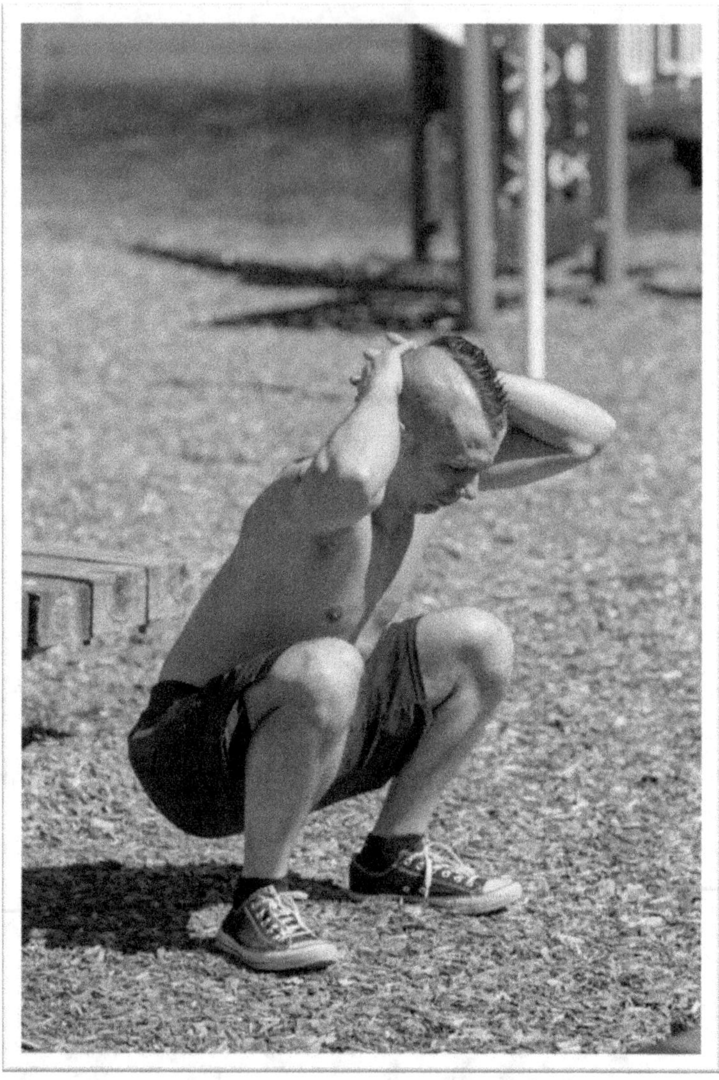

Deep squats takes your butt to your heels, or ass to the grass as some would say. Getting this low will take that little extra flexibility in the knees and ankles, so you may not get there right away, but go as deep as you can and try to push it a little each time. There is debate on the foot placement, however. Some people say feet need to be directly under the hips, others say slightly wider with toes slightly turned out. Again, the best answer I can give is, test it out and feel it out for yourself.

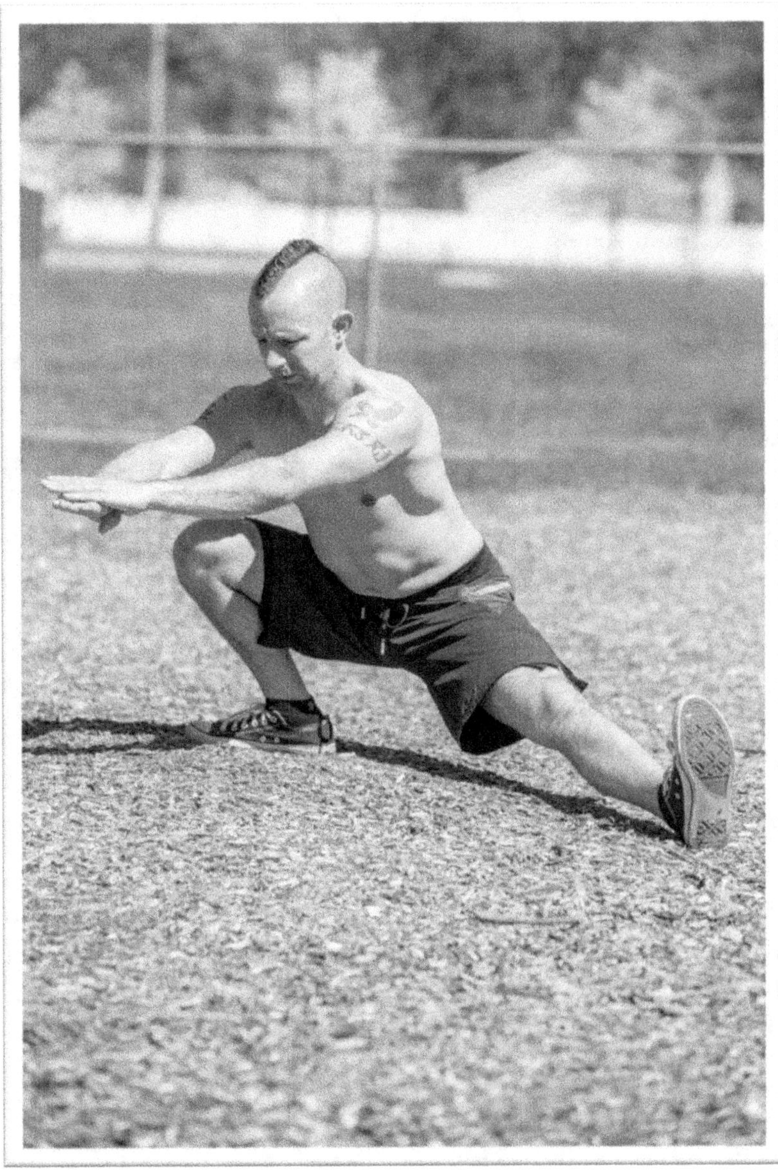

Side Squats are what I would call the archer move for the legs. For this you will need to open your feet a bit wider and squat down to one side straightening the other leg. Like the other archer moves, you may not get that opposite leg straight at first. Be sure to repeat this on the other side.

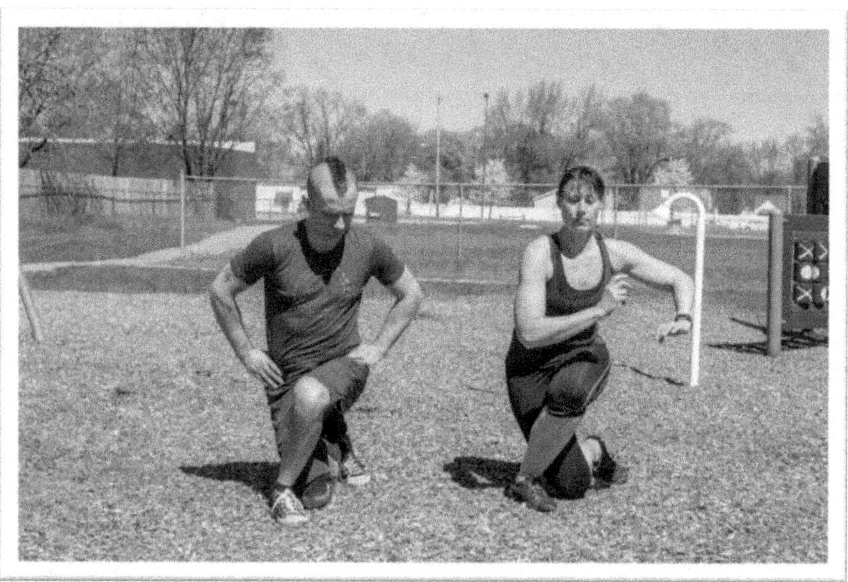

The Curtsy Squat is the opposite of the Side Squat. From a standing position, step one leg behind the other crossing the legs. With the planted leg sink down into your squat, all the way down until the back knee touches the ground if possible. Push back up with the rooted leg, and don't forget to train both legs equally.

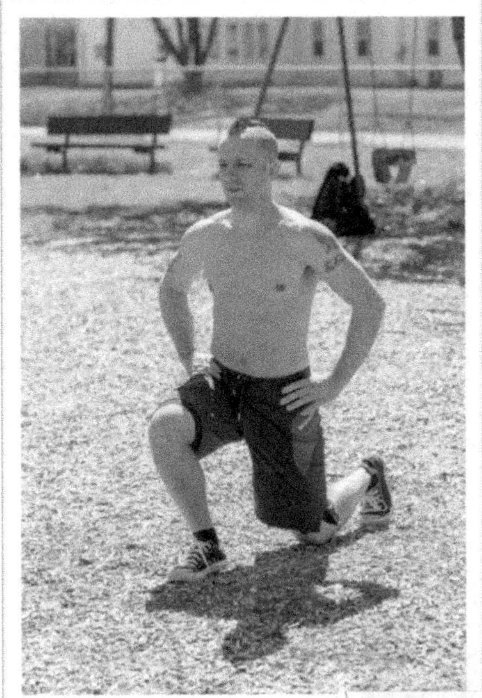

Split squats, or stationary lunges, are another great leg workout. I recommend with this one to play around with the width of the legs as well as how far you have them apart front and back. This will change up the challenge. Remember, without challenge there is no change. Any who, once your legs are in position sink down trying to bend that back leg to 90 degrees, then push back up. Once you finished on one side it's time to hit the other.

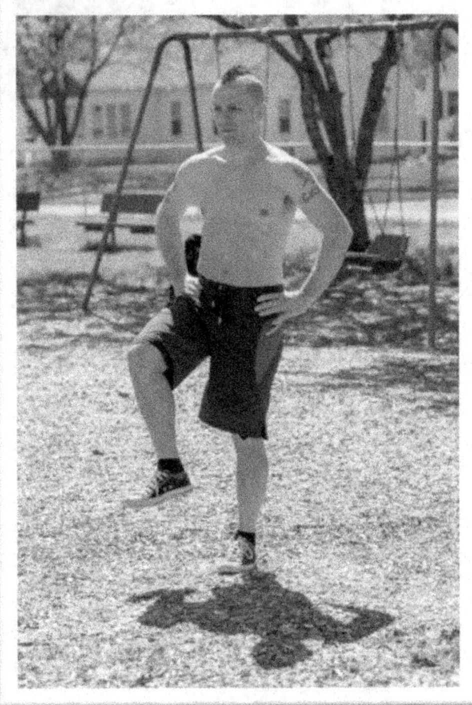

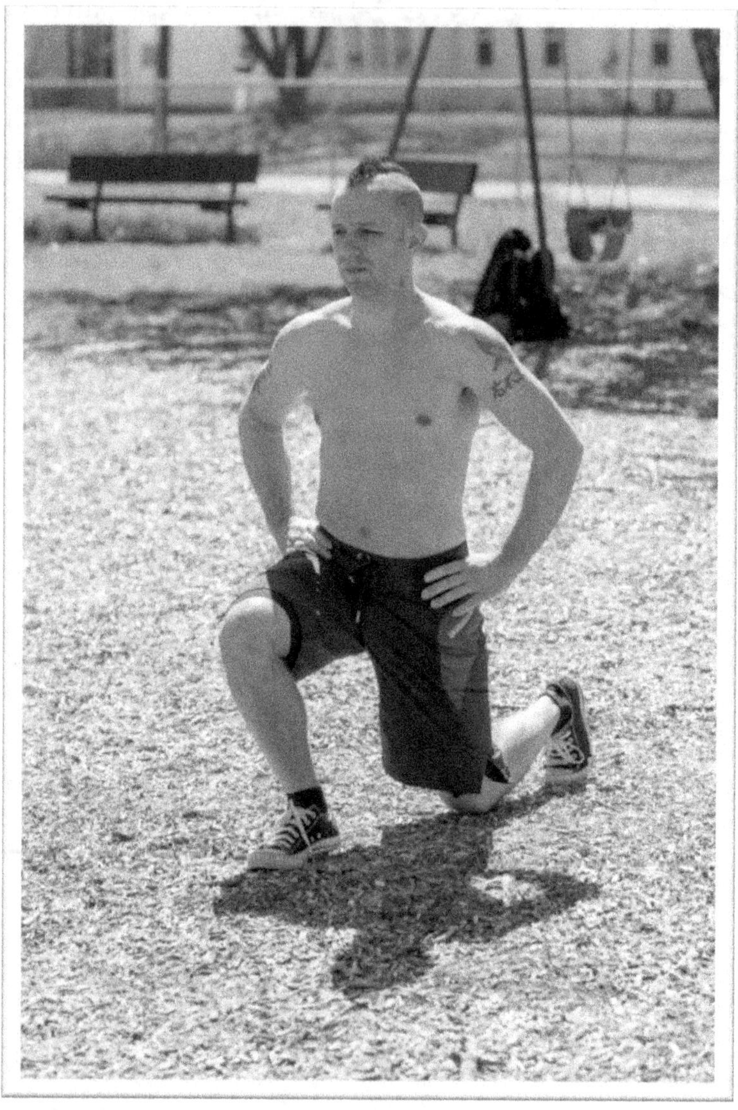

Lunges are another classic move for the legs, and there are a few great ways to do them. First up is the forward step lunge. All you need to do is step one foot forward and sink down trying to get the legs to 90 degrees. The other way is a backwards stepping lunge, this one can be a little more challenging as you are moving backwards.

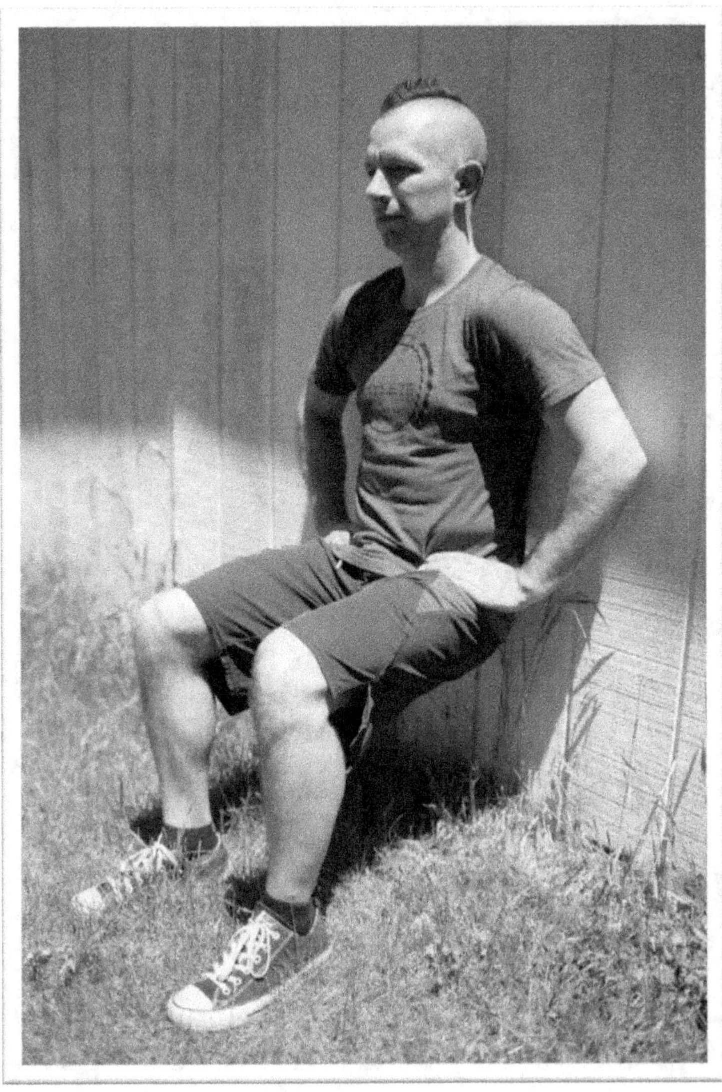

Wall Sits are a fantastic leg workout using no movement. Sure it looks like all you have to do is sit there, but man do those legs burn after a short time! To start lean against a wall or other stable surface, and walk your feet out as your back slides down the wall. Try to get your hips and knees to 90 degrees and your back pressed into the wall. Once here, just hold it.

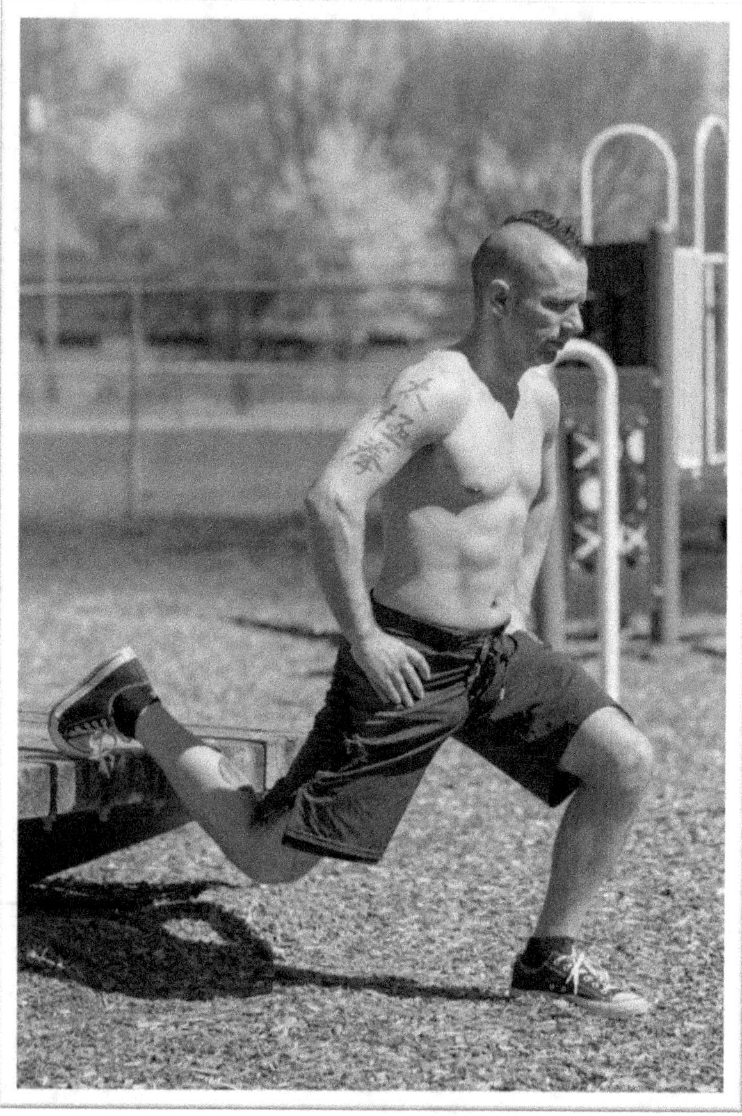

Another great balanced squat is the elevated split squat, a.k.a. the Bulgarian Split Squat. For a lot of heroes out there this one is a challenge. For this you place your back foot on an elevated surface such as a bench, and the other foot on the ground. Once in this position squat down on the one leg. Don't forget to work both sides evenly or you may walk in circles due to one strong leg. Just kidding on that, but you should still do them evenly.

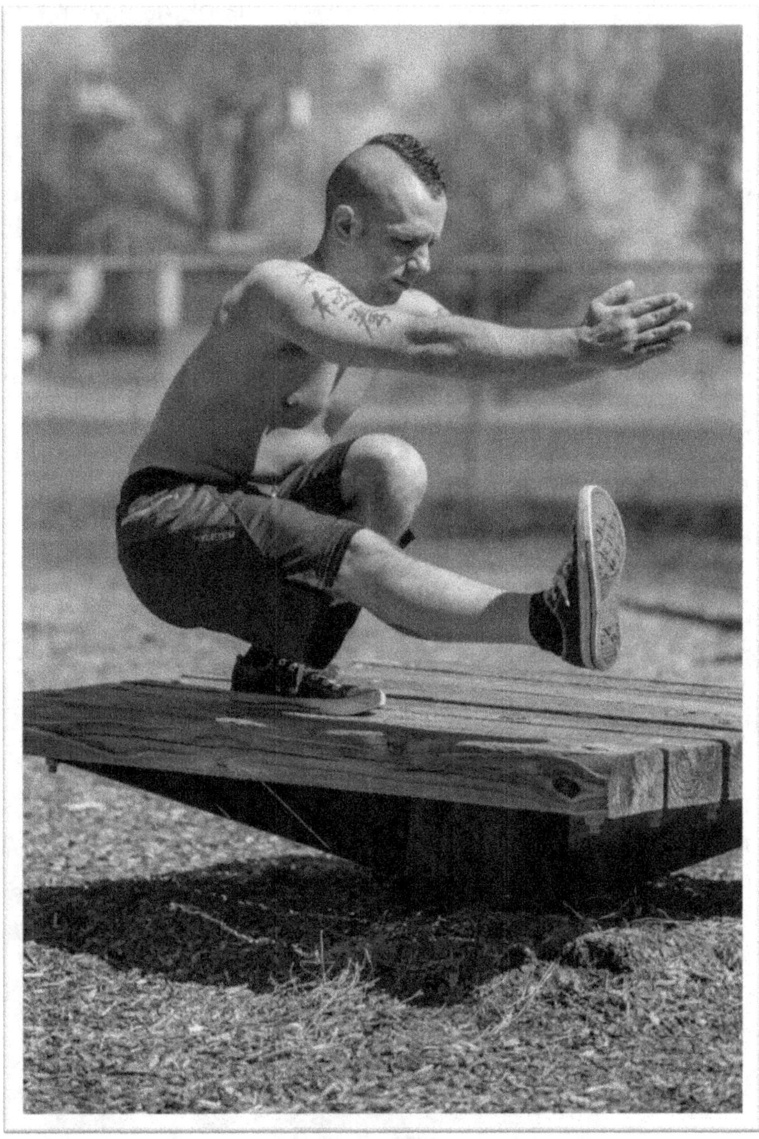

Draw your pistol! Pistol squats are tricky, it requires balance, flexibility and core strength. A classic pistol starts with one foot one ground and the lifted out in the air. Then keeping the one leg lifted you sink into a squat position. I know there will be a lot of hesitation on this, GOOD NEWS! They can be regressed just like regular squats!

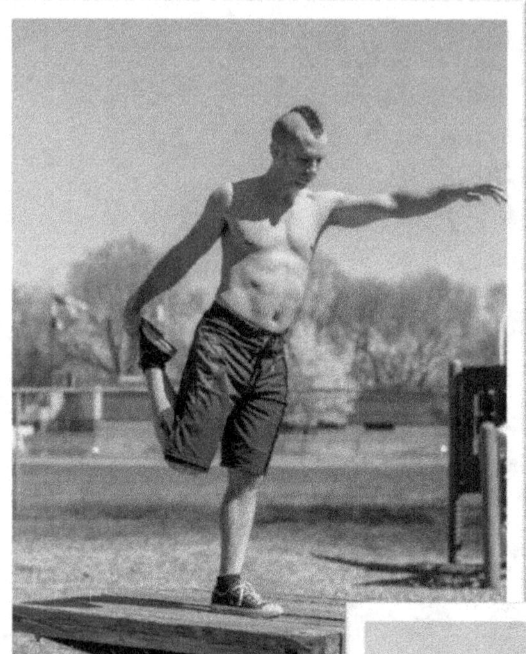

One of the newer squats I like to do is a Shrimp Squat (newer to me, they have been around a long time). This one for a lot of people is more challenging than the pistol. Like the pistol, you are balancing on one foot, but this time the foot that is off the ground is behind you being held with your hand. Your goal is to be able to sink down and touch your back knee to the ground. I would highly suggest putting a pad on the floor for your knee if you are new to these. Smash your goals, not your knees!

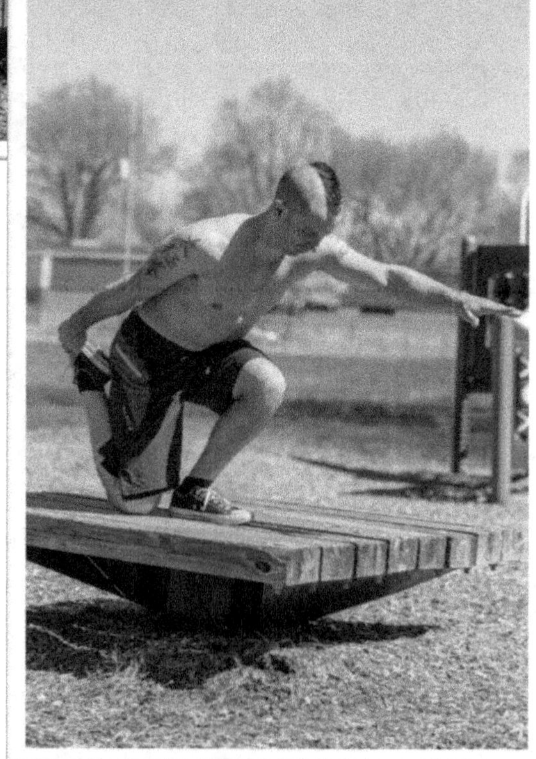

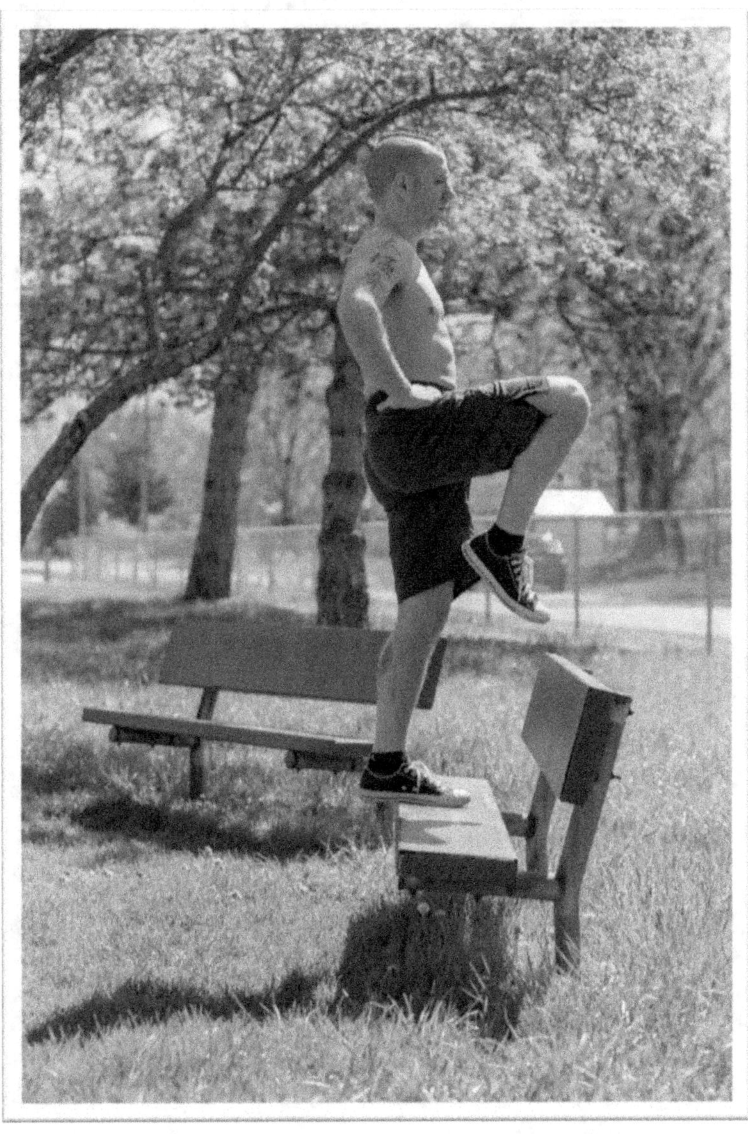

Step ups are great to build up those legs, I use them a lot. Find a sturdy elevated surface, and while facing it place on foot on it and step up just as the name suggests. Try to keep from pushing off to much with the back leg. Let that front leg do the work. After you get the reps in switch legs.

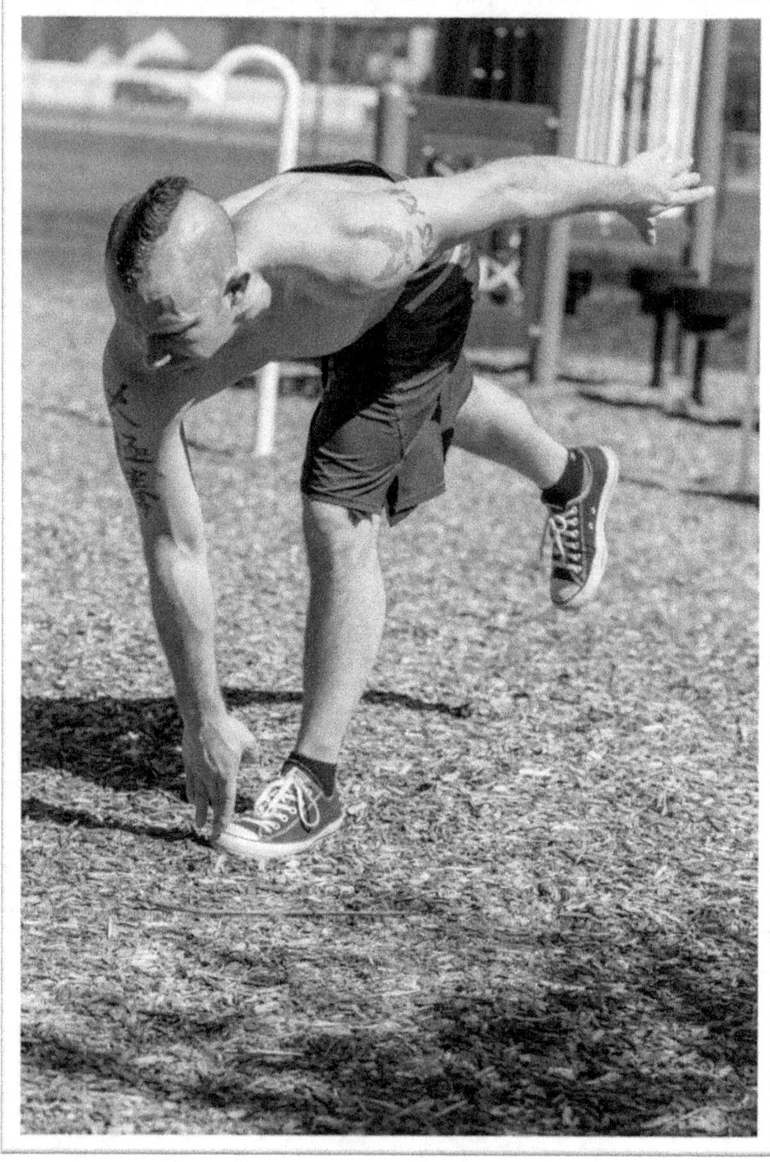

Straight leg single leg deadlifts (I have also seen them called Drinking Bird) can really fire up those hamstrings and the booty. Once again you are balancing on one leg keeping only the slightest bend in the knee. From there bend from the hips and reach towards the planted foot with the opposite hand, then pull yourself all the way back up. Feel the booty burn!!

Chapter 9
Getting Inverted and Skill Leveling!

I can't tell you how much I love hand balancing. But, before we get into it, I would highly suggest warming up the wrists. This can take some wrist flexibility as well as strength. Some gentle wrist bents and wrist rolling is a good way to start. Once warmed up, it's time to conquer the hand balancing. I will tell you, it is a challenge to get use to your hands doing the balancing instead of the feet. Do you have what it takes to control gravity?

One of the first balancing exercises to start with is the frog pose. So to get this one going, get yourself down in the deepest squat you can and place your hands about shoulder width apart on the floor, bend your elbows and rest the inside of your thighs on top of your elbows. Gently slide your weight forward and slowly bring one foot at a time off the floor. At first you may only get one foot lifted, but it's a start!

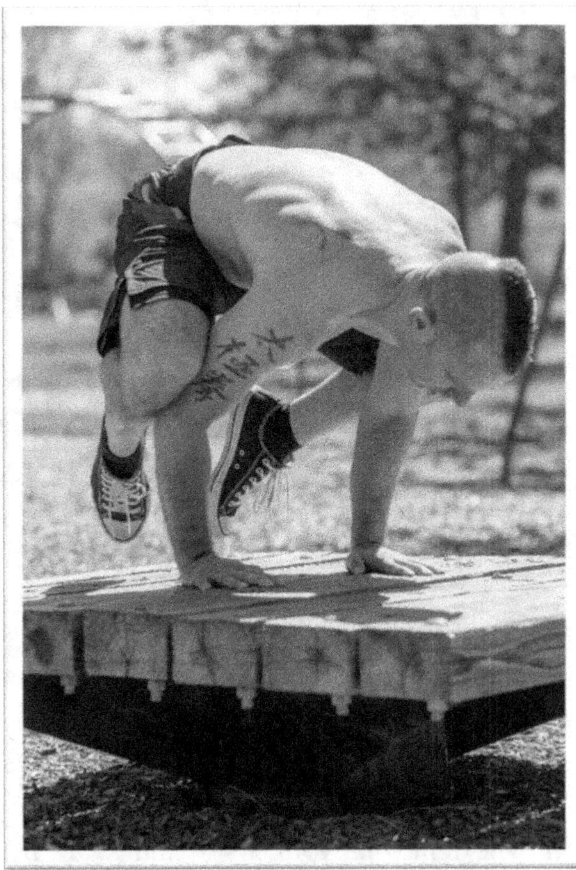

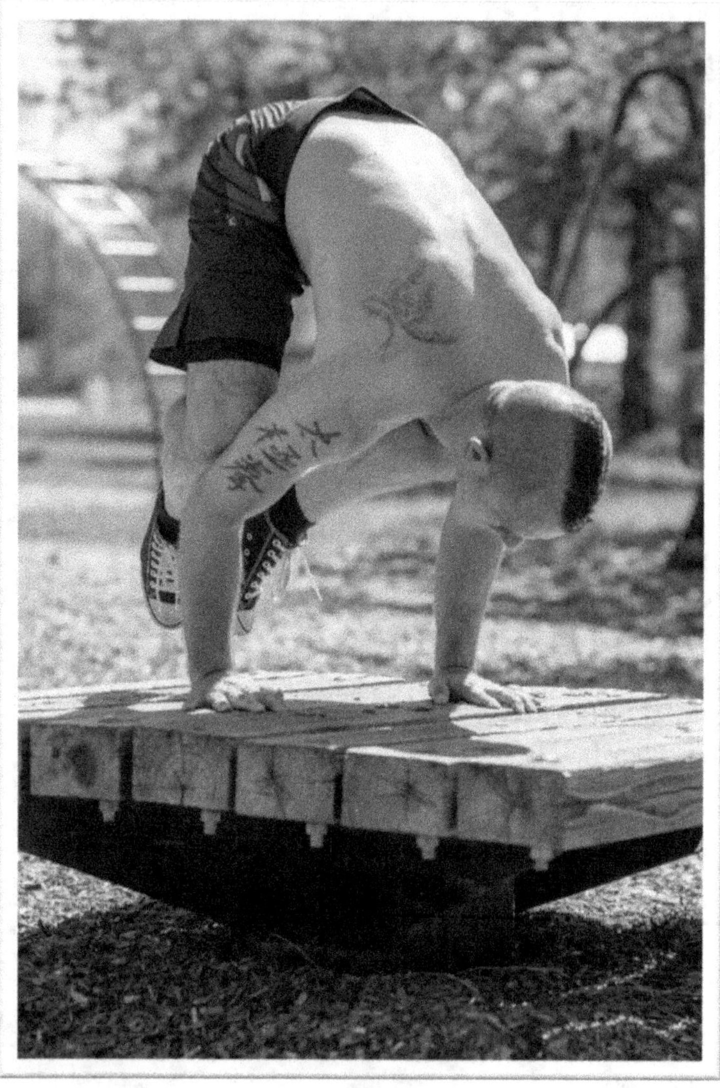

The Crow is similar to The Frog, yet it is a different animal. (See what I did there?) Similar to the frog, you start at the bottom of the squat with hands on the ground. This time place your knees on the back of your triceps and slide the weight forward. Again, once foot may not be able to leave the ground at first. Once you are balancing in this regularly try to straighten out the arms. This will for sure test the flexibility in your wrist and your balance. There are other variations to the crow, such as single leg crow and twisted crow.

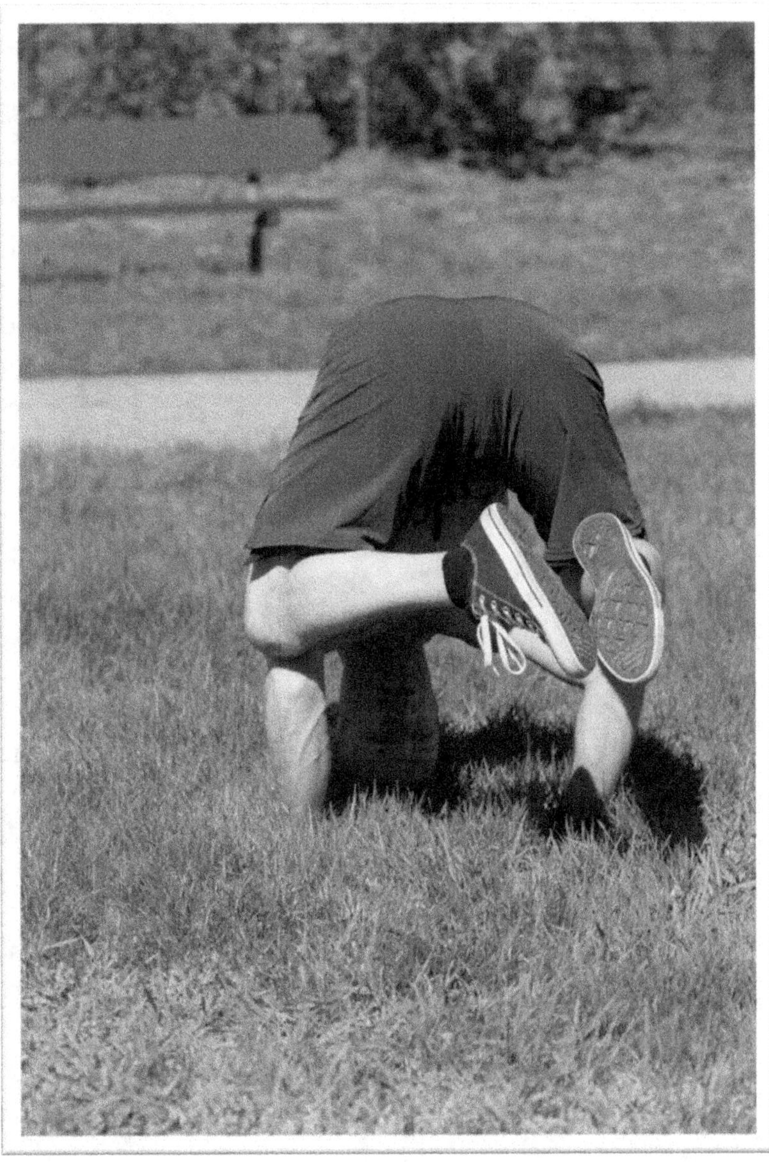

Now it's time to get inverted. The first big step is the tripod. Getting to the bottom of the squat, hands on the floor as well as your head. From there bring the knees up onto your elbows and your feet go up to the sky. This may be a challenge at first, but keep working at it, you will get it.

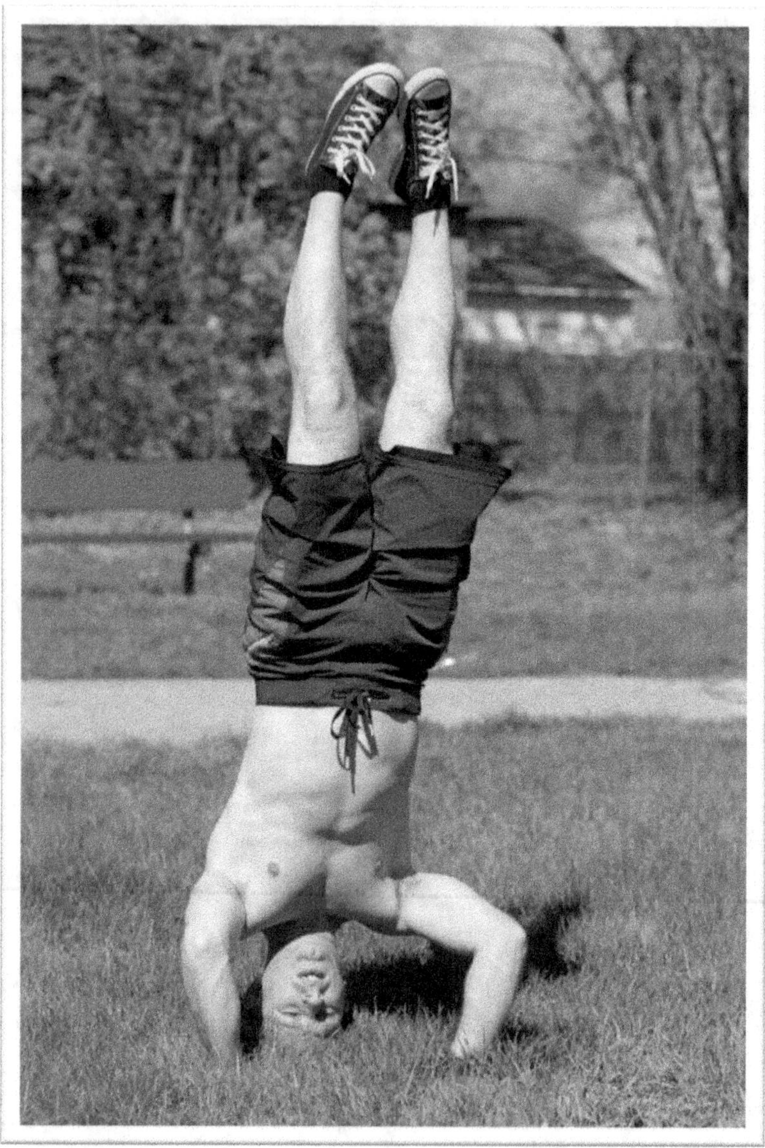

So, you hit the tripod, now it's time to go skyward with the head stand. Start off the in that tripod you nailed down. Once balanced, extend your feet all the way up. I would suggest at first to do this close to a wall or with a friend to spot your legs. The first full inversion will feel a little wobbly.

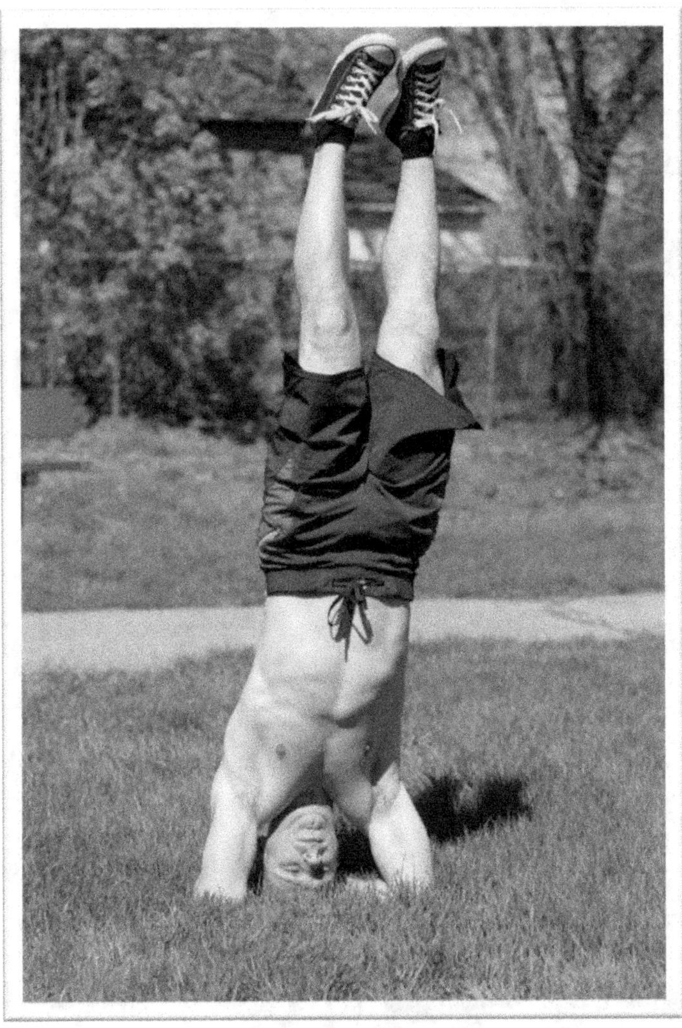

The elbow head stand, other than looking rather awesome, is the next challenge. It is challenging in a few ways. First, you can't really start off in the tripod so you will need a little more core control. Second, it will take a little flexibility in the shoulders since you are balanced on your forearms and elbows. In this experiment, I would suggest getting the head and forearms on the ground and extend the legs up one at a time. At first you may have to kick the legs up to get inverted. Once again, a wall close by or a friend would not be a bad idea just to brace you a little.

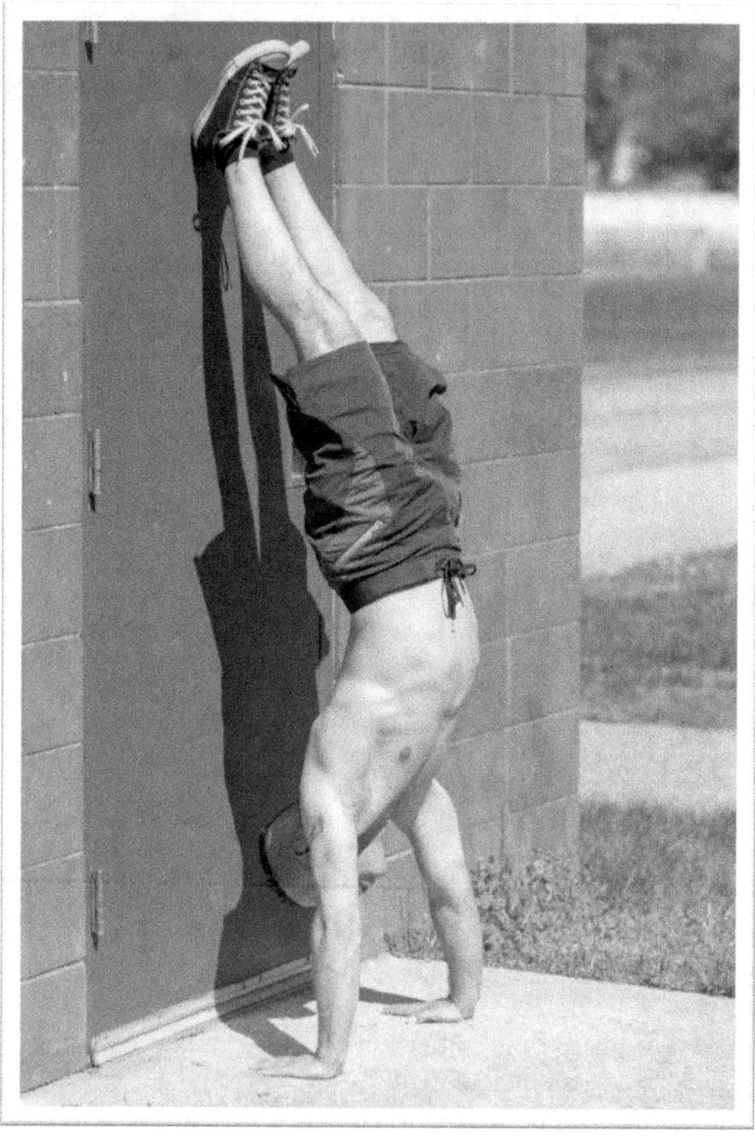

Hand Stands are the next big level up. At first that transition may not be smooth, but we all have to start somewhere. There are a few ways to start and the first one is to use the wall. Walk your feet up the wall as you walk your hands closer. Once you are comfortable getting inverted, it's now time to try kicking up to the wall hand stand.

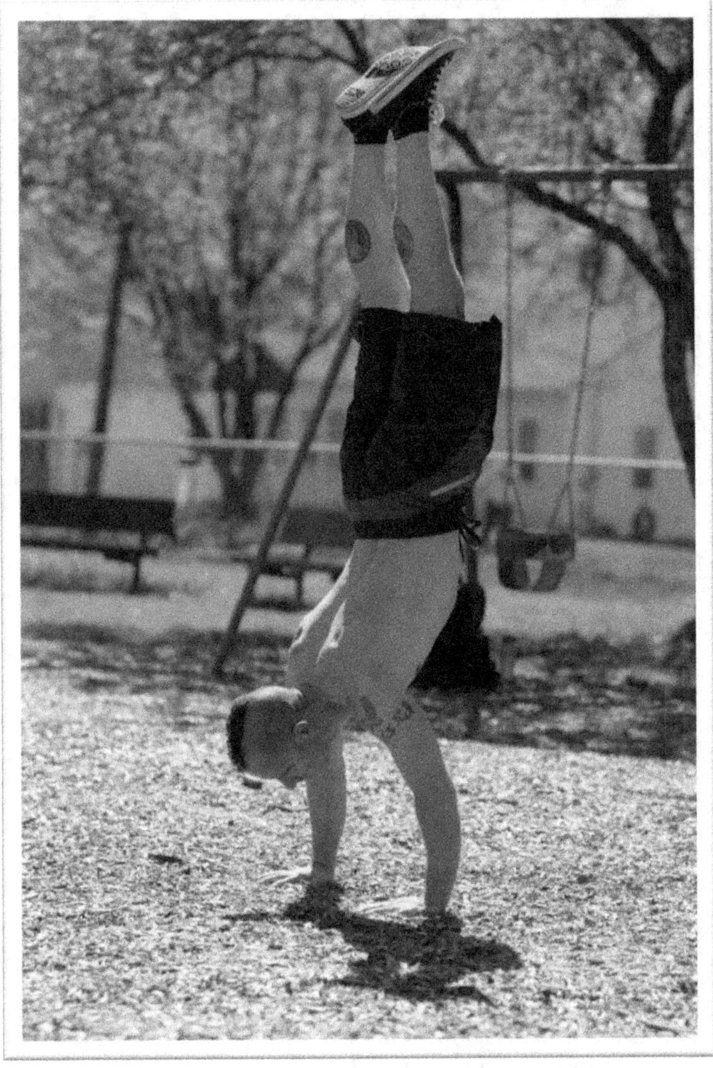

Free standing hand stands are not easy, but they are impressive when you have them down. Few ways to get into it, the first is to kick up next to a wall and start removing one leg from the wall at a time. When you can hold it, try to move away from the wall and ease into it. One way I like to train it is to move from that Crow Pose to a hand stand. This will take a lot more shoulder and core control but it is well worth it. Learn to control your muscles to master your universe.

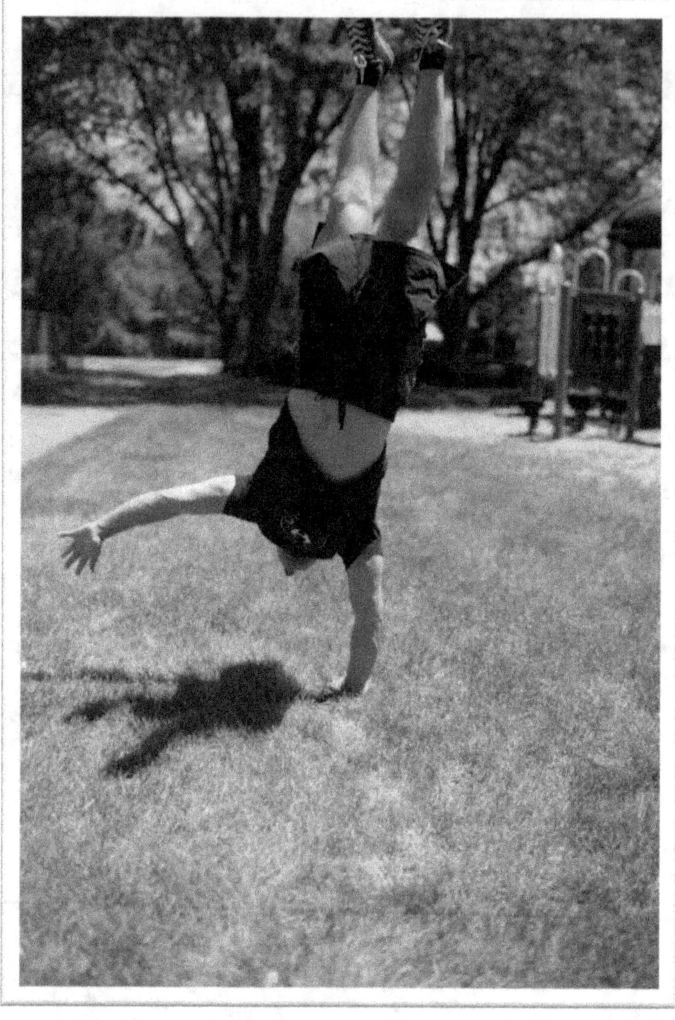

One Arm Handstands are insane and take a lot of practice and shoulder strength, but if it doesn't challenge you it doesn't change you and this is all about going super powered. Using the wall for stability is advised, and don't be afraid to try it both forward facing and back facing the wall. Once you are up into your hand stand, straddle your feet and start shifting your weight over to one arm. At first you may need to keep a few fingers on the ground, and slowly remove them. When it feels like you have the balance take one hand all the way off the ground. Be patient! This move will take a lot of time, and even more to go free standing.

Chapter 10
Balance on the Elbow

Elbow Levers are by far my favorite hand balancing move, and people love to see it! It's almost like flying, in my world. To hold your body parallel to the ground with your hands is a true feat of strength. This will take balance and power and core strength. When you start out I would suggest an elevated surface, such as a bench this will give you something to grab on to. Once you have it down you can do it anywhere.

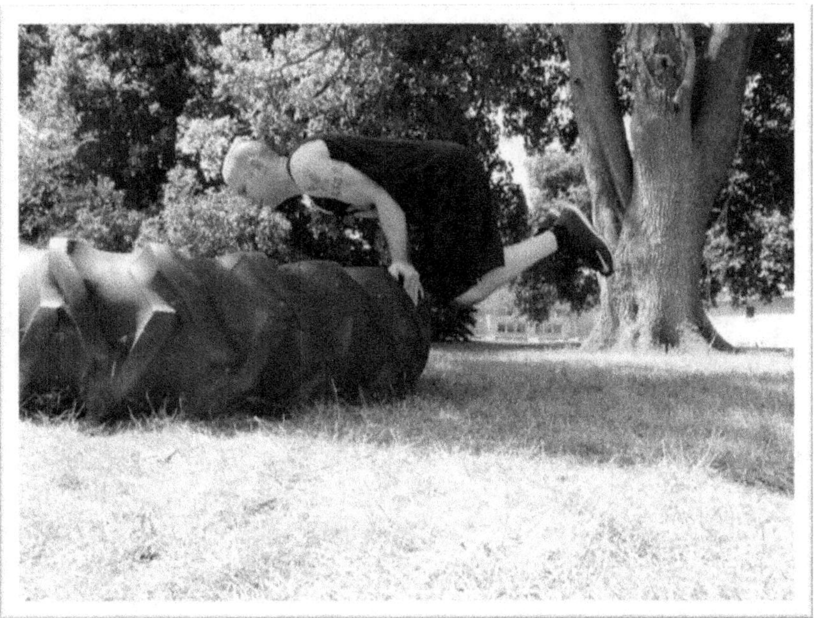

A Knee Tuck Elbow Lever is a great way to start and to learn that body balance. This one will need that elevated surface we talked about. Place your hands on the elevated surface with fingers pointed towards you and not far apart. Bend your elbows, bend your body forward and lay your abdomen on your triceps. Slowly take your feet off the ground by slowly shifting your weight forward and hold your core tight. For now just keep your kneed bent while you work on this balance.

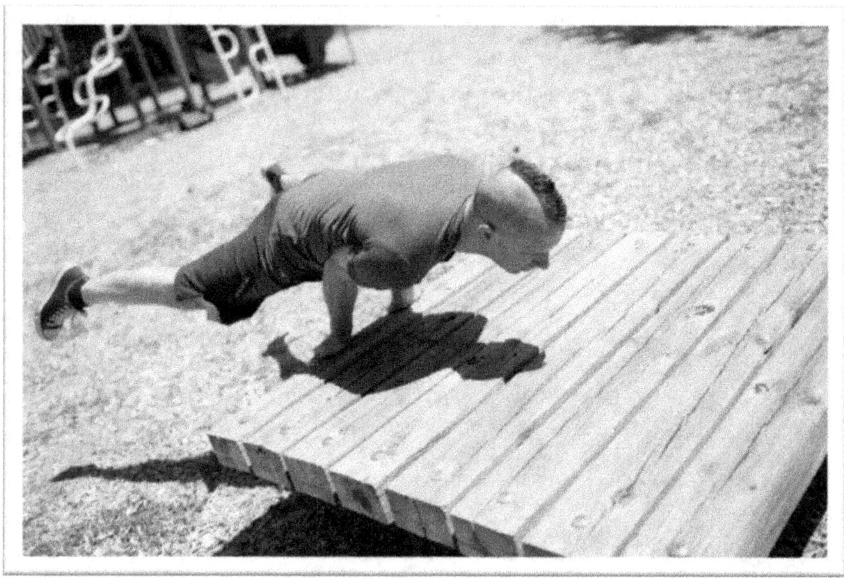

Straddle Elbow Lever is next, once you are comfortable with balancing your body on your elbows. Get into that balanced Knee Tuck Lever and slowly extend your legs out in a V shape while slowly sliding yourself forward, your arms have to be a bit further than 90 degrees.

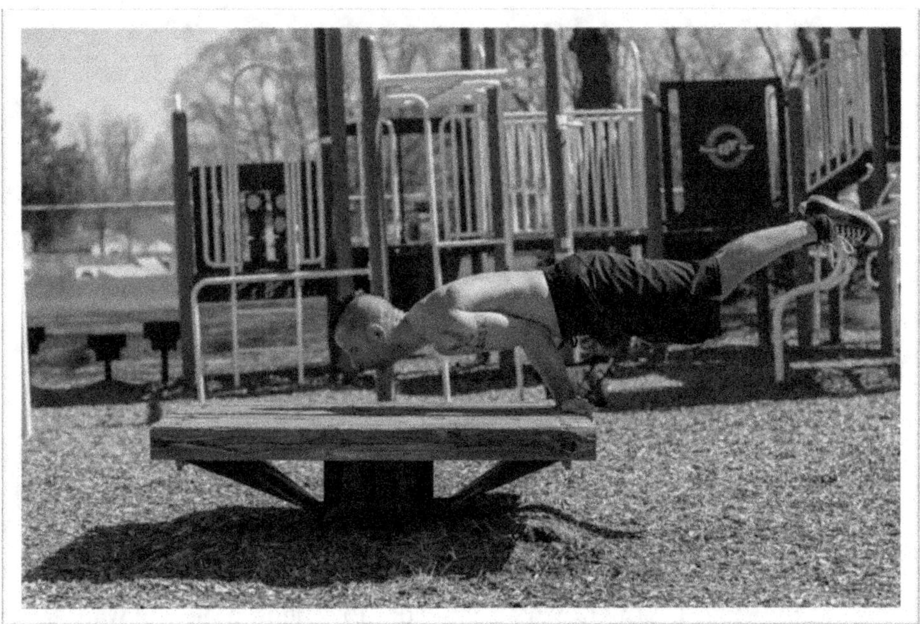

Elbow Lever is finally here! Once you are up in that Straddle Elbow Lever and your confidence is up it's time to bring those legs together. Make sure to keep your body tight to keep your back flat and legs straight. Remember that your body needs to slide forwards a bit to keep that balance point.

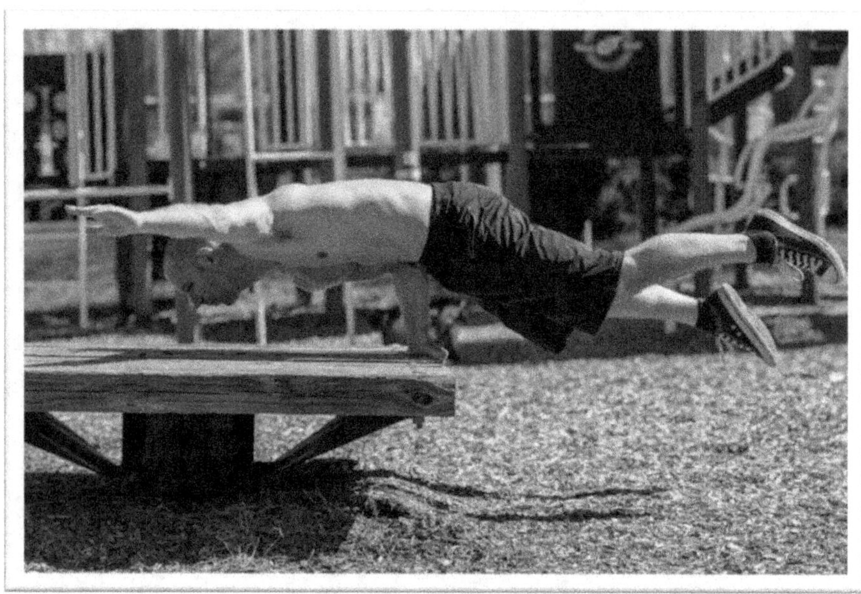

One Arm Elbow Levers are a true boss fight. You will want to get into that Straddle Elbow Lever, now that you are here slowly extend one arm out. For now keep the hand on the ground, and find that balance on the one elbow. There is a chance you may have to slightly tip to one side. Once you have an idea where the balance is, one finger at a time remove that extended hand from the ground. You will find one side is stronger than the other, but work to even the arms out.

Chapter 11
Going to the Bar

Bar Skills take all you have learned in your Planks, Pull-Ups and Push-ups and kicks it up to a crazy level. Yes, these bare moves are awe inspiring and epic to see, but there is a lot more than cool looks. All of these moves will take practice, and persistence they will not come over night. Through this you will learn to further bend the laws of gravity.

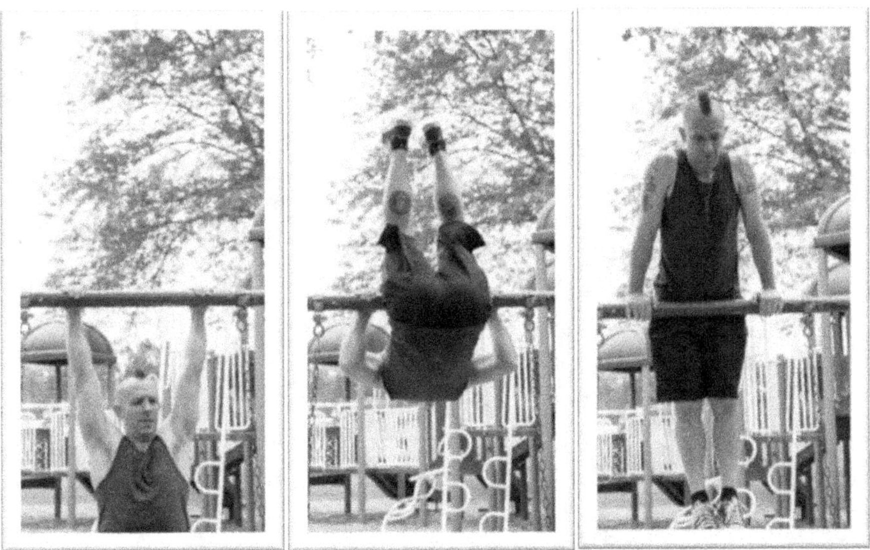

The Pullover is a great way move to train many other bar moves such as the muscle up or straight bar dip. To get it under way, grip your pull up bar and bring your toes up to the bar like you are doing a toes to bar leg raise. Start pulling until your hips go over the bar. While you are pulling the hips over the bar you will start to invert. Kick your hips over the bar until you roll over the top.

Magnificent Muscle-Ups

Muscle-Ups are one of the most fun moves and one of my favorites. It looks like a mix between a pull up and a dip, but it is far, far more. This move requires explosive power, core control, pulling and pushing all in one move. But there are a lot of steps to get to the top of the bar world. First up, you need to be able to get at

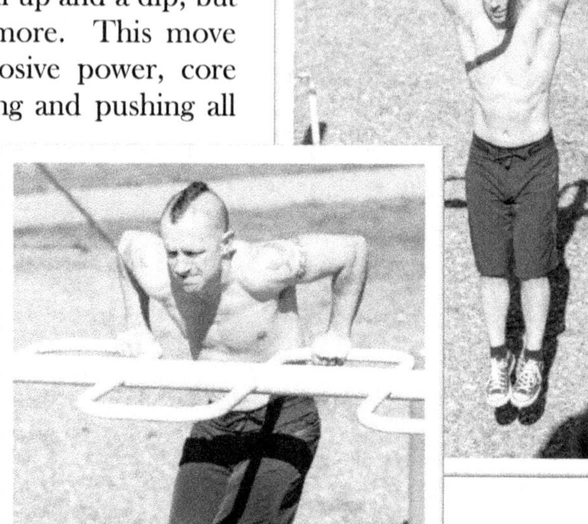

least 10 strict and deep pull-ups that means full control with no kipping and getting the bar to your chest. Next up, you need to be able to get about 20 straight bar dips. Now you need to work on explosive pull-ups, pulling fast so your hands can almost leave the bar. When ready, start at the top of the bar and work the negative muscle-up. That means get to the top and lower yourself down slow. When you're ready, it's time to try the muscle-up. Odds are it will not be pretty, but it's a start. Start at the bottom of the bar and pull yourself up with a lot of power and fold yourself over the bar rolling your hands to the top. When here push yourself up with a straight bar dip. I know my first one wasn't great, and I tried many times before I even got an ugly one.

Face Up to Front Levers

Front Levers may be one of the harder bar hangs you will face. But like everything else, if you are determined enough you can beat this one too. It's like flying but with your back to the ground. It's going to take strength in your core, arms, legs and the rest of the body to hold yourself level to the ground. But let's start from the bottom.

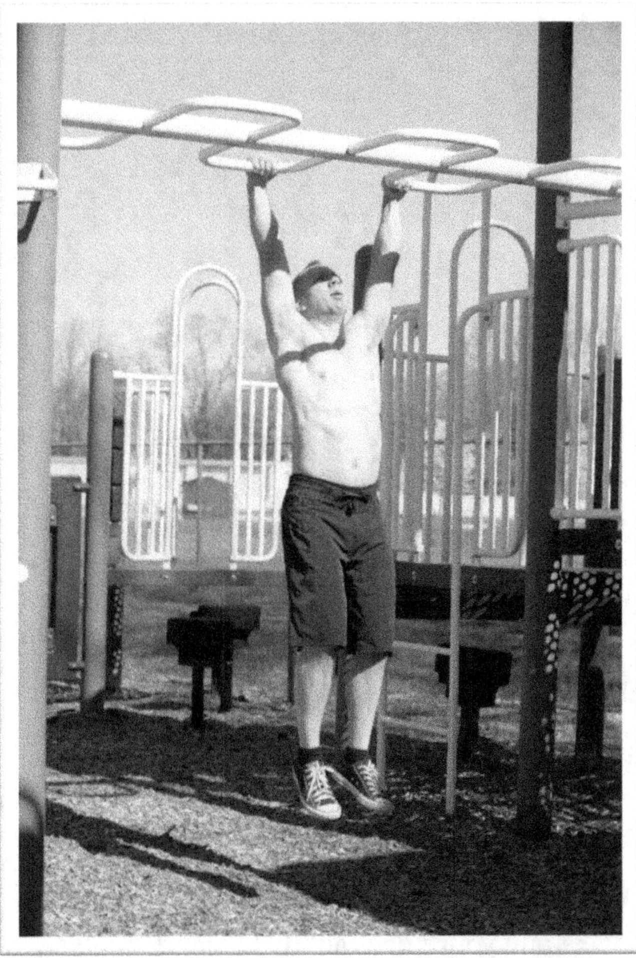

Bar Hang is a great first step to learn how to control your core for the Front Lever. It's almost like planking while hanging from a bar. Grab a low bar and extend your feet out, now pull your shoulders down and back and tighten your abs. While holding this squeeze your shoulder blades together. Keeping your arms straight, imagine pulling the bar towards your hips and hold it. Try to do this without bending your arms. Another option is to put your feet on an elevated surface. The next step is to do this while hanging from the pull up bar.

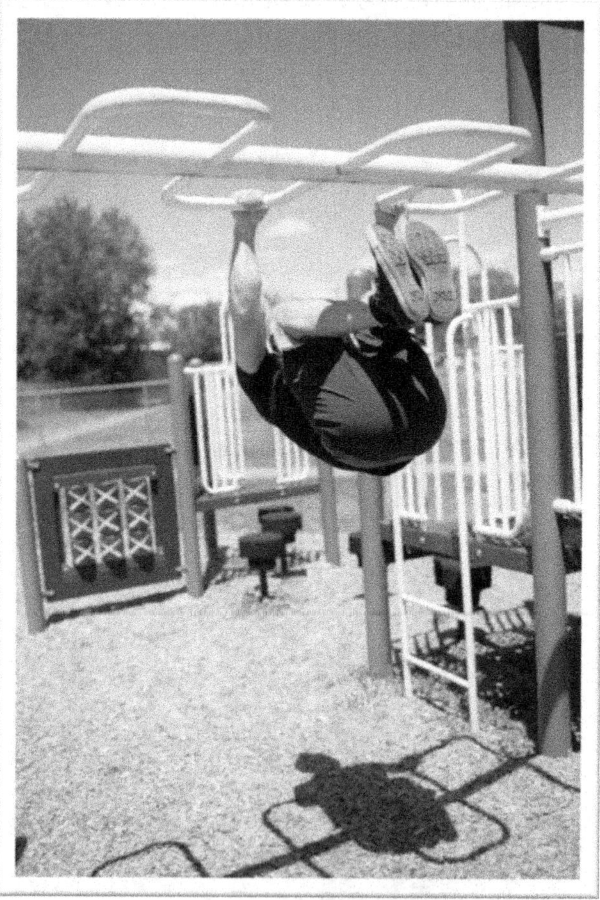

Tuck Front Levers are next stage in the lever evolution. Grab onto your bar and tuck your knees towards your chest. Once your knees are all the way up, start rolling back pulling the bar towards your hips making your back parallel to the earth and engage your back muscles. The more tucked un your knees are the easier this will be to hold.

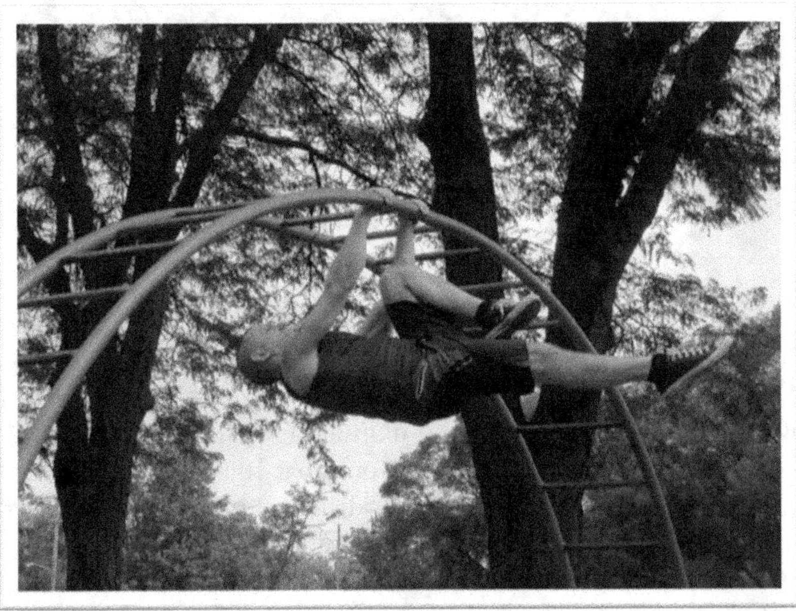

Single Leg Front Lever Takes the Tuck lever up to the next level. Pull your knees up to the tuck position and tighten your core up just like in the prior regressions. Once in positon, slowly extend one leg out straight. You may not be able to hold it long but that's ok; it's a start. Remember to train both sides.

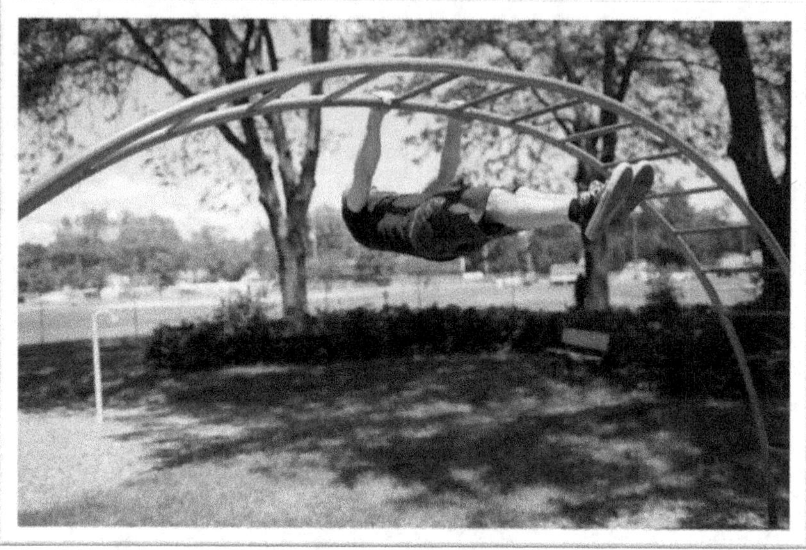

Front Lever time! So, you can hold the Single Leg Front lever for a bit now, so let's take this to the ultimate levels. So, there are a few ways to attack this one, and the first one that I used was a front lever swing. This is done by swinging the body up to the lever position from a hang position and holding for a moment and lowering back down but this is a harder method. This can be done for reps. The second way is to go into the tuck position, and extend your kegs up and slightly invert yourself, and slowly lower yourself down to parallel. The final way is to start tucked and slowly extend your legs out to a hold. You will need to generate a lot of tension throughout this movement.

Back Levers Take Flight

Back Levers get you facing the earth. Just like the front levers, this will take some full body strength as well as some grip strength. You will want to condition your shoulders to get here. Like so many other skills, there are a lot of levels of progressions to go through to train you up to it. Ready for the challenge of flight?

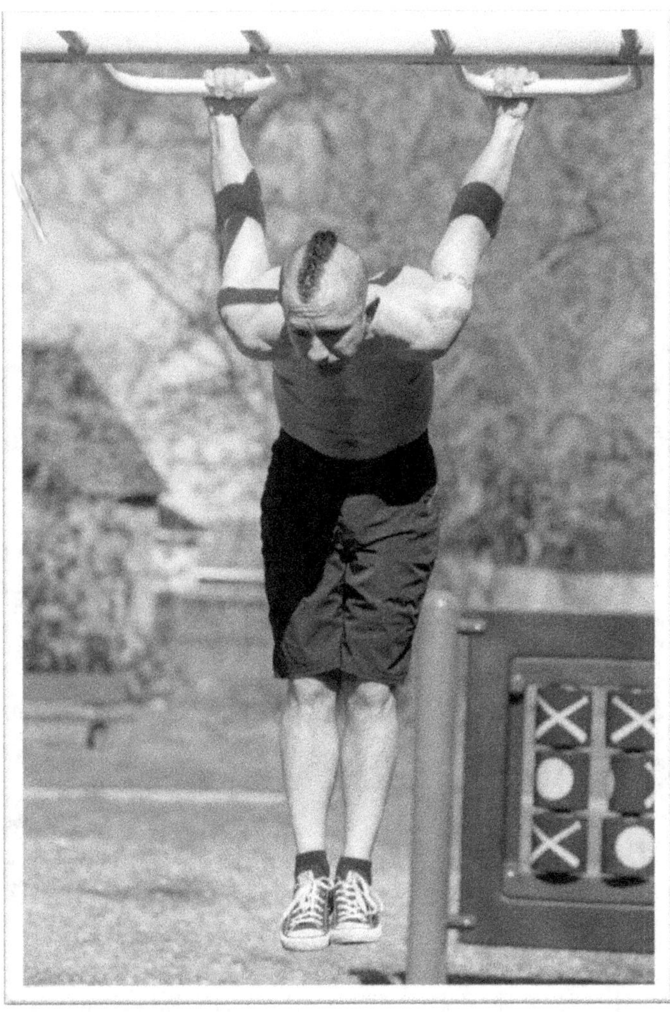

Skinning the Cat is not as horrible as it sounds, and has nothing to do with a cat. Now that we got that out of the way, grab the straight bar, putting yourself in pull up position, and tuck your knees into your chest. Once they are as far as they can go, begin to roll your body and legs under the bar until you reach the other side. When you get there lower your legs down towards the floor while your arms are behind your back. While in this position you will feel an epic stretch in your shoulders. Hold it here for a moment, this position is also called a German Hang, tuck your knees back in and rotate back through. As your flexibility increases, you may be able to pass under the bar with straight legs.

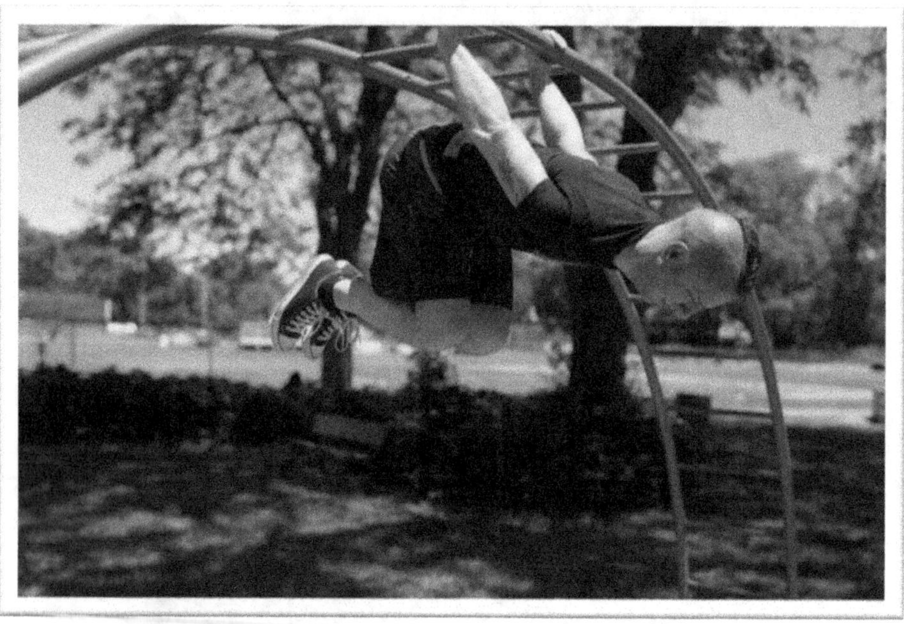

Tuck Back Levers are a starting point to work into the Full Back Lever. Start by working your way into the Skin the Cat to the German Hang. Lift your knees towards your chest and flatten your back. Try to get your body parallel to the ground. Really concentrate on not rounding your back.

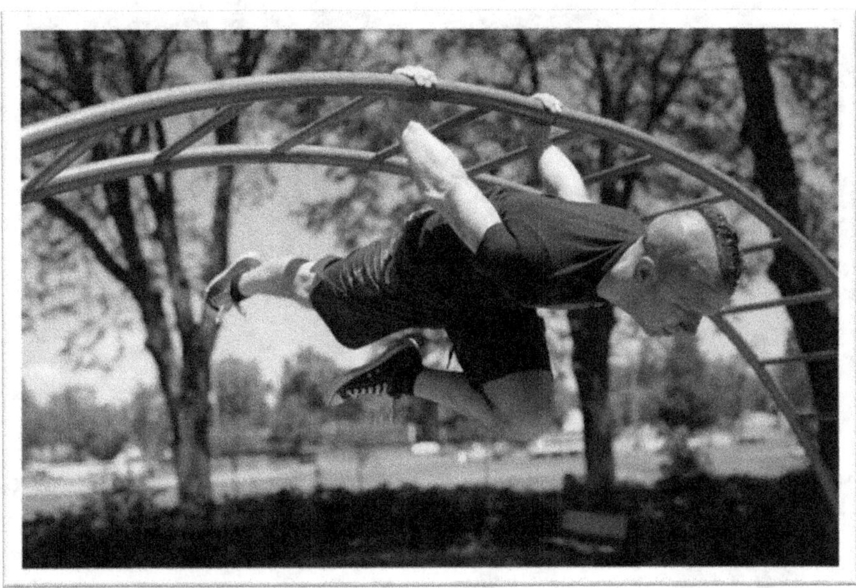

Single Leg Back Levers bring you a little closer to the real deal. Get into the German Hang, then tuck your knees in to the Tuck Back Lever position. Slowly extend one leg out keeping the other tucked. In this position, you will feel an increase in the tension throughout our body. Try to hold it for even a few seconds, but make sure, like always, to train both sides.

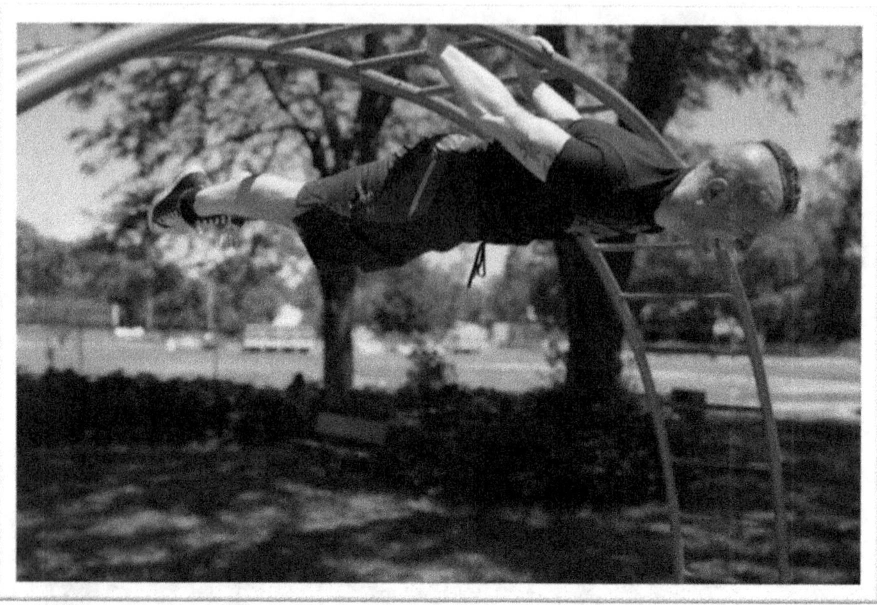

Back Levers are your path to flight in this super hero quest. They will not be easy, and they will not happen right away, but when you get them they will draw a crowd to your skill. This will take a lot of body control, grip strength and a full body squeeze. I highly suggest to use the steps that came before to build you up to this. One of the ways to get into position is to start in the Knee Tuck Back Lever and extend your feet skyward as your head lowers towards the ground. At this point, you will be inverted on the bar. From here you can attempt to lower yourself down until parallel to the ground. The other method I have used is to get into the Tuck Back Lever, then slowly push both legs out finding your balance as you extend. What every method you choose, make sure to engage your lower body, glutes, and all the rest of your core muscles. Think of it as a downward facing hollow body. This is another move where you can play with the grip a little when you have it down. You can work wide, narrow or even a reverse grip. If you do try the reverse grip, it will put a lot more stress on your biceps, so make sure you have the foundation down first.

Chapter 12
Flying Your Hero Flag

If the Muscle-Up is a demonstration of strength and power, then the Human Flag is the demonstration of epic strength and control. At no point will I tell you that flags are easy. You will want to train the hell out of your shoulders and your entire core border lining becoming superhuman to do this. Even the first stage flags are hard. Now this isn't to dissuade you from trying them, I just want to make

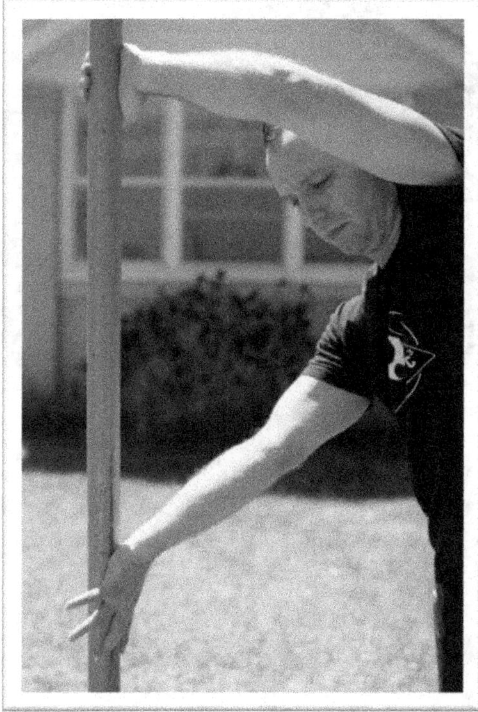

it clear that they are an epic challenge, but with proper training you can crush them.

One thing to work on, before you even get started, is just working on hand and body placement. This will be key to your successful flag. First off let me say your bottom arm will be your foundation and main support, so start with your strongest arm on bottom. With the bottom arm grip the bar with the fingers pointing towards the ground. Now lock the arm out with the shoulder lined up with the bar. With the other arm grip the bar overhead using the pull up grip. Without even lifting your body up, just practice pulling the bar with the top arm and pushing with the bottom, almost like you are turning a gigantic wheel. If the bottom elbow bends or the shoulder doesn't line up then you may not catch flight.

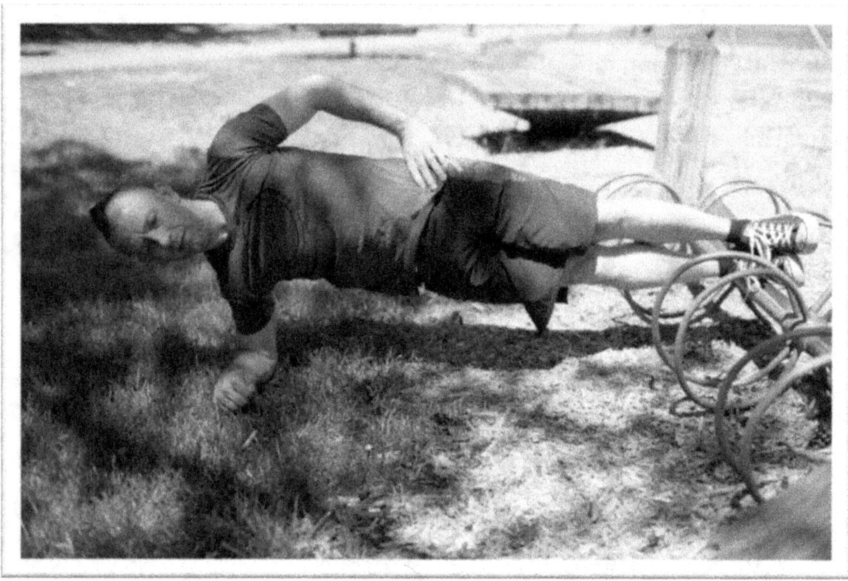

Elevated Side Planks are one of the methods I used to work into Flags. Start off by getting yourself in the side plank position. These can be done on the elbow or straight arm. Once in position, place your feet on an elevated position and engage the core.

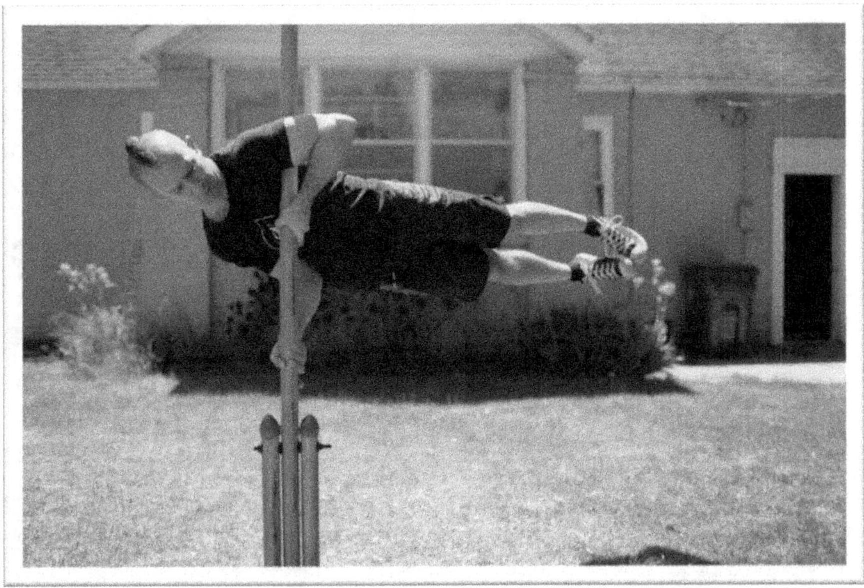

Clutch Flags are your next flag step, and it oddly feels like you are putting the bar in a crazy headlock, with that said, you will not be extending your arms straight out but you will still be working to get parallel with the earth. There is a chance you will not get your legs straight out at first, but try it even with your legs tucked. Now onto the steps for your clutch flag. First thig first, pick a side to try it on. With the hand that is going to be on bottom. With this hand grip the bar at about waist / hip height with your thumb pointing towards the ground getting as much as your palm as possible on the bar. Then, lean into that arm getting your chest close to the bar. Now, with your other arm wrap it around the bar as if you are putting it into a headlock and squeeze it tight to your chest. From here, try to swing your legs up to become horizontal and tighten all your muscles. There are a few options if you can't get them all the way straight. Try them with knees tucked or with your legs angled a bit towards the ground.

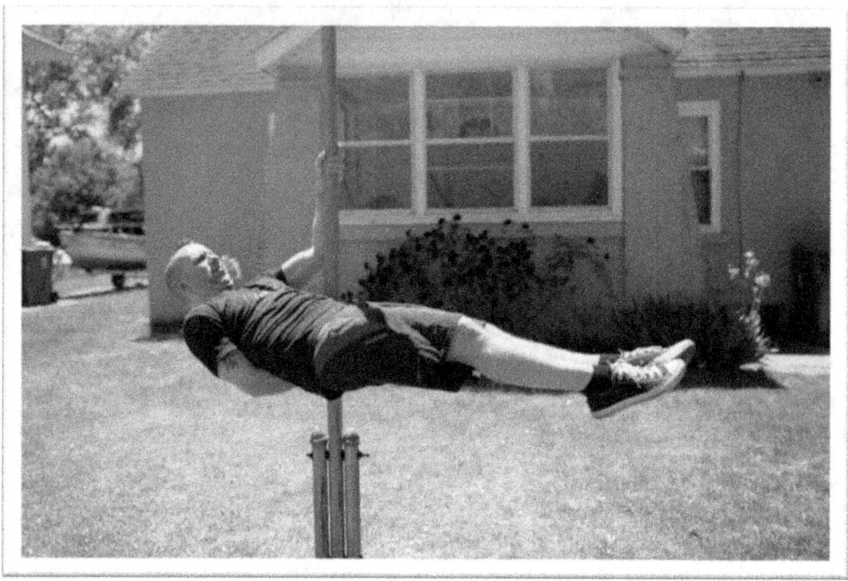

The Lever Flag or Clutch Lever is another one I like to play around with. This almost looks like something you see in a magic show. To start, stand with your shoulder next to the pole and grab the pole with the hand closest to the pole at about chest height. Next, reach behind your back with the other hand and grab the pole at about waist height. Lay back on the arm behind your back looking for that balance point, tighten up your entire body and extend the legs out flattening out the body. To keep from spinning out of control, like a super hero being knocked out of the sky, try not to lean against the bar.

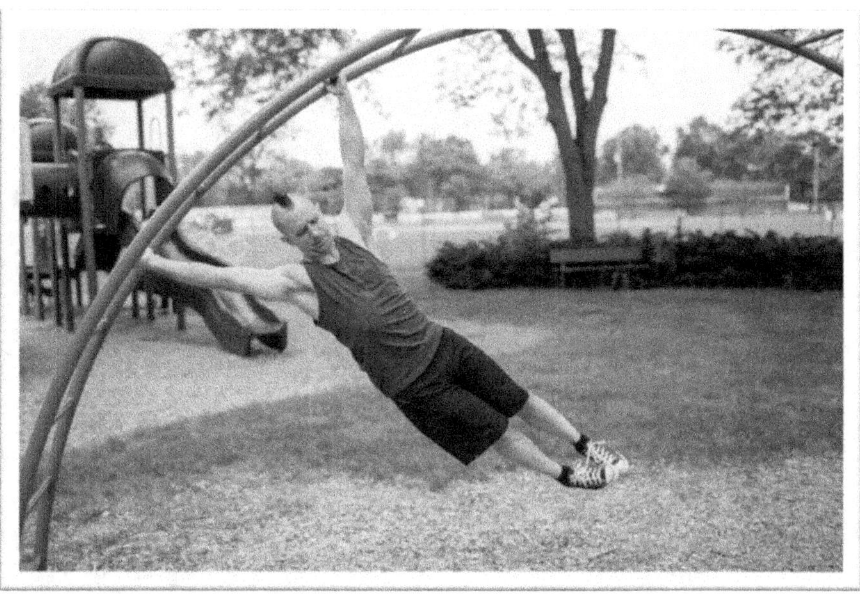

Angled Flags a.k.a. Support Press are a great way to work into your full flag. Now, this will put a lot of tension in your shoulders and core, so no worries if you can't hit it just yet. To start grip the vertical bar with your strongest arm with your thumb again pointed towards the earth. Make sure to lock this arm out and line your shoulder up with the bar, if you don't then you will collapse in before you even really start. With the other arm grab the straight bar overhead. From here press out with the bottom arm and pull up with the top arm and tighten your core. From here angle your body out keeping everything from your shoulder to your ankles engaged. You should be trying to hold at about a 45 degree angle. You may only hit it for a moment, but all you need at first is that one moment to be a super hero. As you get stronger you can press yourself further from the vertical bar.

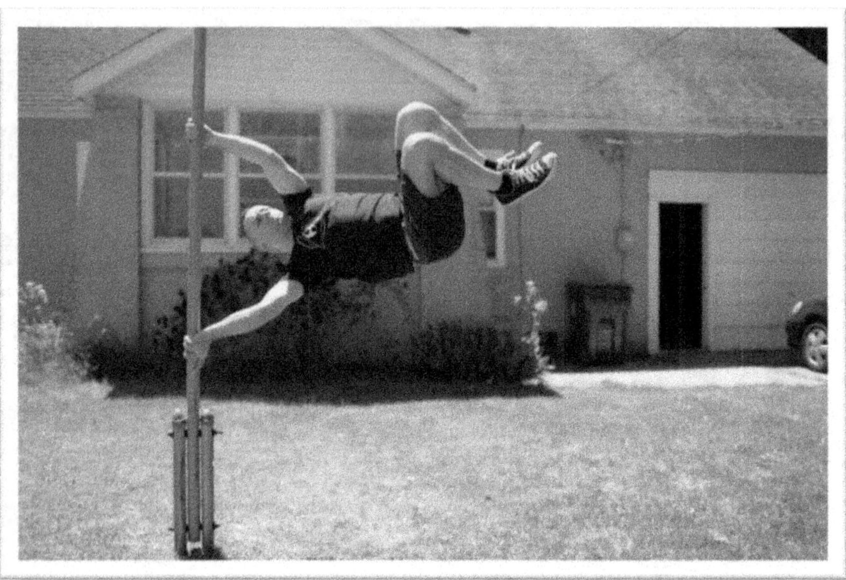

Tuck Flags will be the first to get your arms into that press flag position. Using the hand positioning mentioned in the beginning of the flag section engage the bar. Now you may have to kick your legs up with a lot of gusto to get into position. So swing your legs up and tuck your knees in to shorten the length of your body. Also, feel free to try to over shoot your target to get into position. You will however still feel a lot of tension in your shoulders and you may not get it right away, but give it a shot... if you feel ready.

Vertical Flags get you to expand out from the tuck, but upwards. Getting into the Tuck Flag first, then slowly push your feet to the sky. At first you can work on just extending one leg at a time. You may just do it with one leg to get started and switch legs in the second attempt. This will be a core killer.

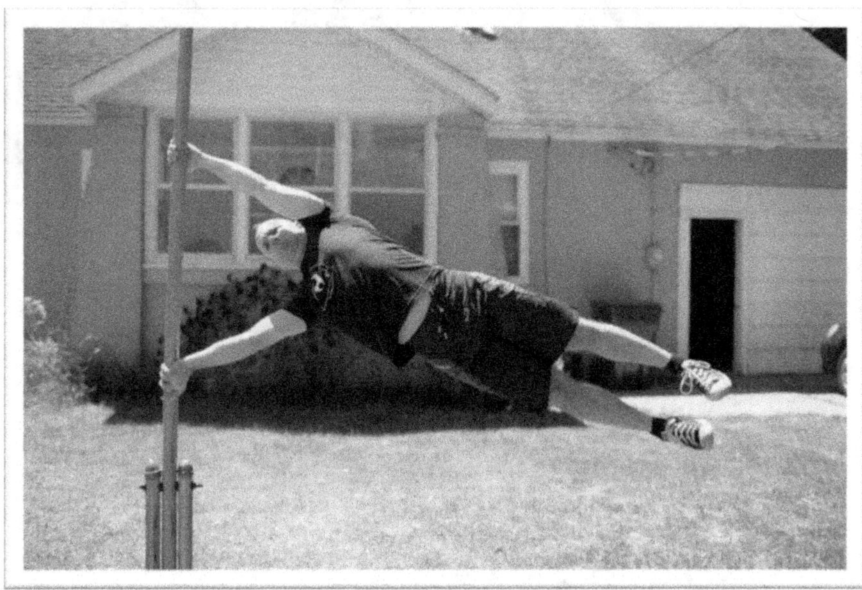

Low Angle Flag is almost the opposite of the Vertical Flag. Getting your hands set up in the press flag position, slowly press the bar with the lower arm and pulling with the upper arm, tighten up the entire body and bring the feet off the ground. In this position, your feet will hang a bit below the shoulders. To be honest, I personally had an easier time with this one than I did with the vertical flag, so as always experiment a little.

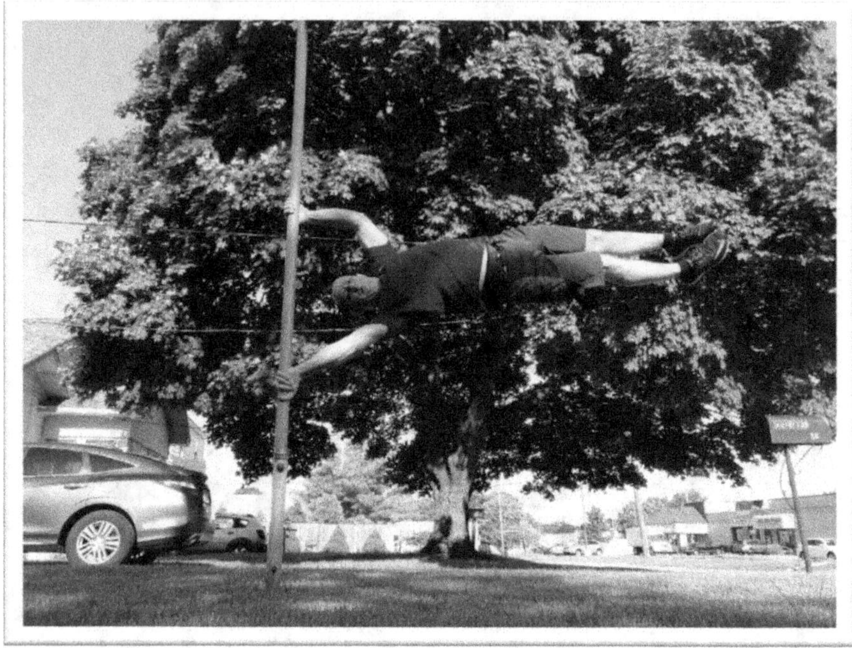

The Full Human Flag or The Press Flag is the king of the isometric moves and exceptionally impressive. Before we really get start, I want to tell you this is harder than a boss fight you are in no way prepared for. It is going to take epic strength and body control, after all you are suspended horizontally by just your hands. With that being said, there are a few ways to work into this once you have your hands and body into position. The first way is to start from the bottom and press up. This one I found difficult to do. Another way is to swing up to the vertical flag and lower yourself down until you are parallel to the earth. The way I used most is to work into the knee tuck position and extend the legs out straight into the horizontal position. Even if you only hold this for a few moments, that is an epic accomplishment. Be proud of what you have done here!

Chapter 13
You have them, but now it's time to get the abs to show!

First, let me say, with calisthenics, every day is ab day if you do it right. There are so many great ab workouts out there and I'm sure you know a lot of them, but let's still uncover them. The most important step to uncovering those abs... The food you eat! Please revisit the nutrition section if this is unclear. Through this we will cover a lot of the basics and even some stuff you may not know. First thing first, keep training that hollow body, you will need it.

Crunches are probably the most well-known ab workout. Just in case they are new to you, start on the ground with legs bent and feet flat on the ground and back pressed down. From this position curl your torso up bringing your elbows towards your knees then lower yourself back down.

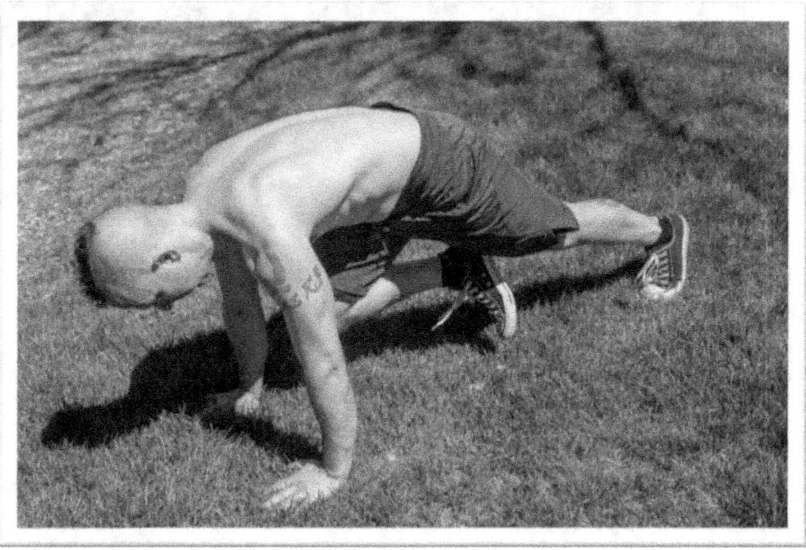

The Mountain Climber has become a staple in my personal workouts. Start off by getting into the High Plank position and hollow your body. From here alternate bringing one knee at a time in towards your chest keeping your butt down the entire time. This can be done fast or slow.

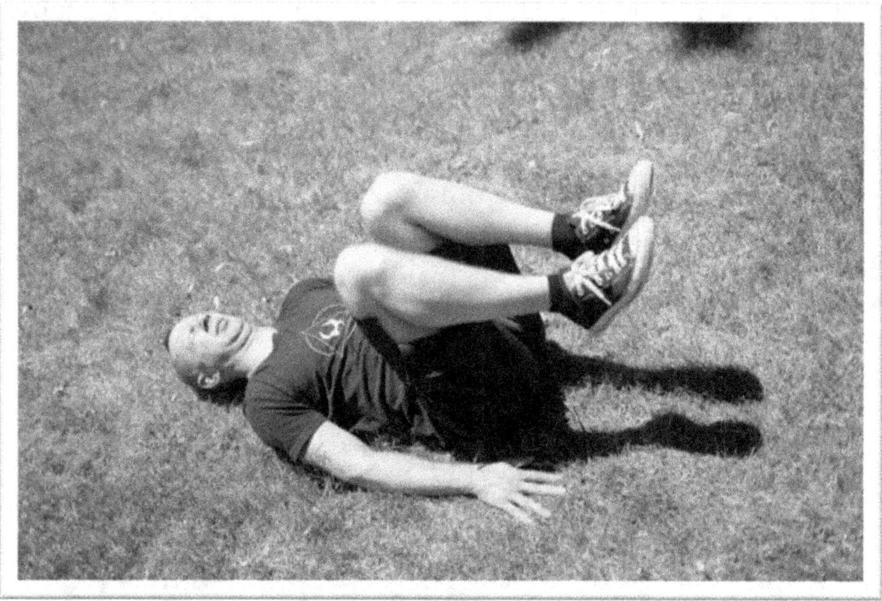

The Laying Down Knee Raise starts with laying on your back with knees bent and lower back pressed into the floor. Once in position bring your knees into your chest and carefully lower them back down. Try not to change the angle of your knees throughout the movement.

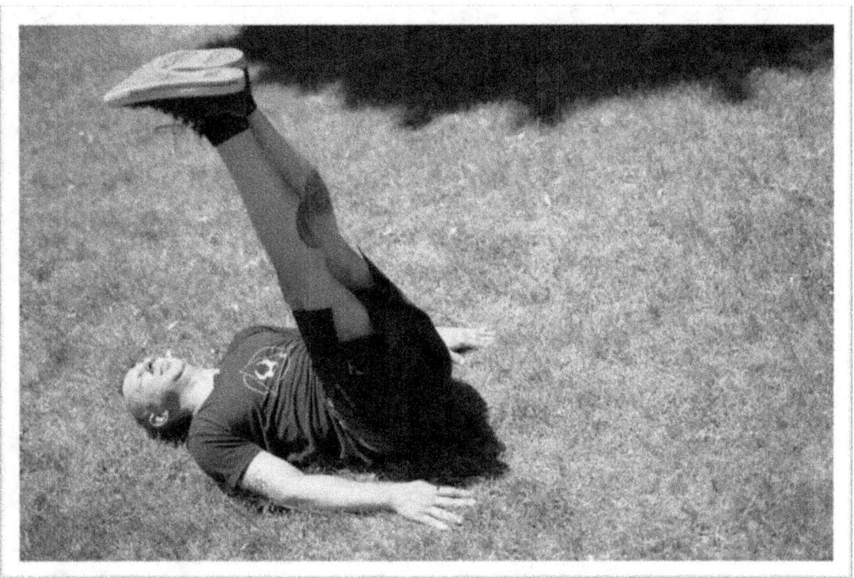

Laying Leg Lifts are an upgrade from the laying knee raise. Like the knee raise, start by laying on your back with your lower back pressed into the floor and legs out straight. Now that you are here, lift the legs up to 90 degrees and lower your legs back down towards the floor. Try keeping your feet from touching the floor.

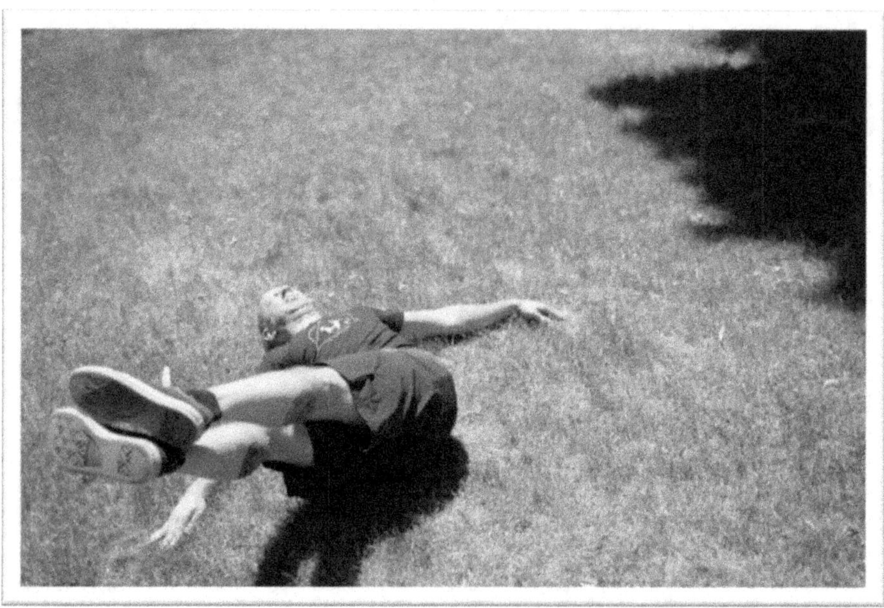

Laying down windshield wipers are like the leg raise, but with a twist, in a literal way. On your back with lower back pressed, lift the legs straight up and lay your arms out to give you a little extra stabilization. From there lower your legs side to side without lifting your shoulders off the ground.

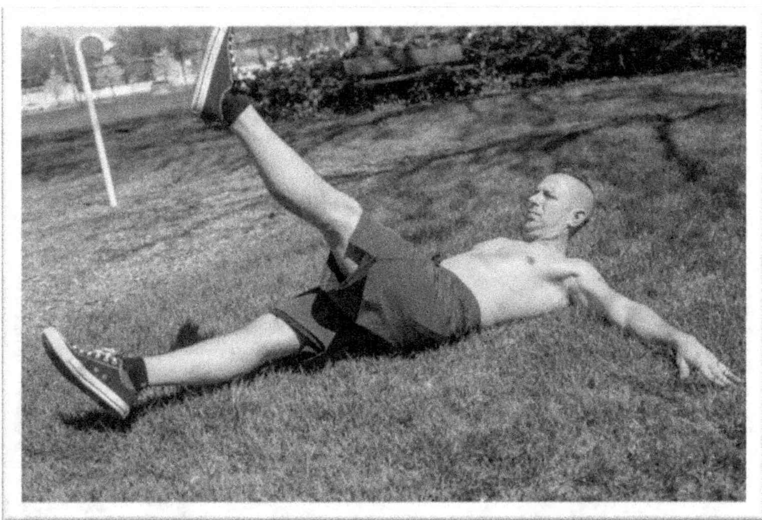

Flutter Kicks sound cute, but they are monsters! Start with laying on your back with your lower back pressed to the ground. Keep your legs as straight as possible and lift them a few inches off the ground. From here alternate kicking your legs.

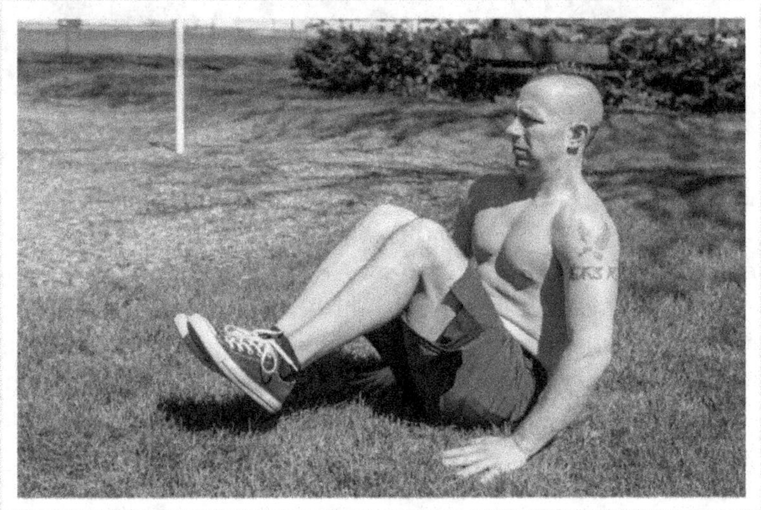

Sitting Knee Tucks start with either sitting on the ground or a bench using your hands on the ground or the edge of the seat. Extend your legs out and tuck them back into your chest. Try to do all this with minimal movement in the upper body. This will be a challenge.

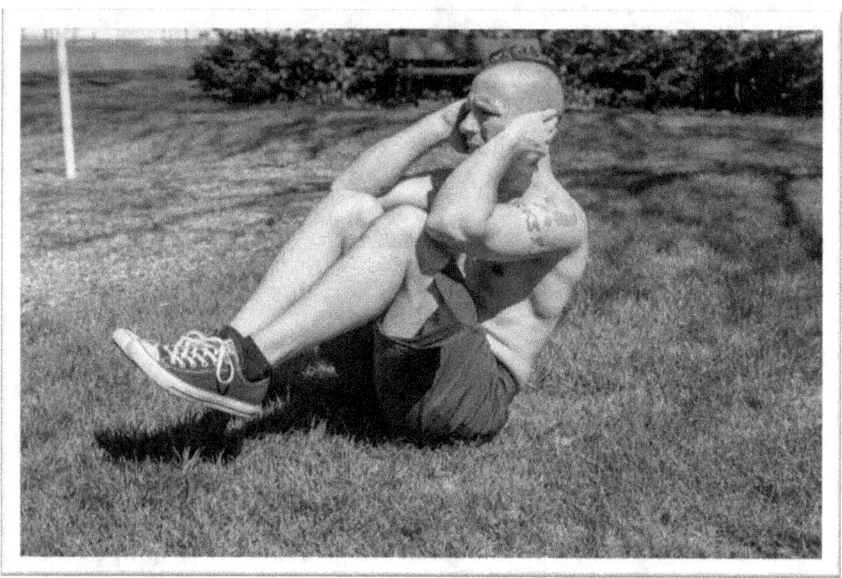

There is a mix move that I call a Tuck and Crunch. Starting off lay on the ground with legs straight and lower back pressed to the floor. From here lift your legs off the ground and bring your knees in towards your chest like a knee tuck, at the same time crunch your body up and bring your elbows towards your knees. Don't worry if you can't get all the way up, be patient. Then, lower yourself back down and straighten out your legs without letting them touch the ground.

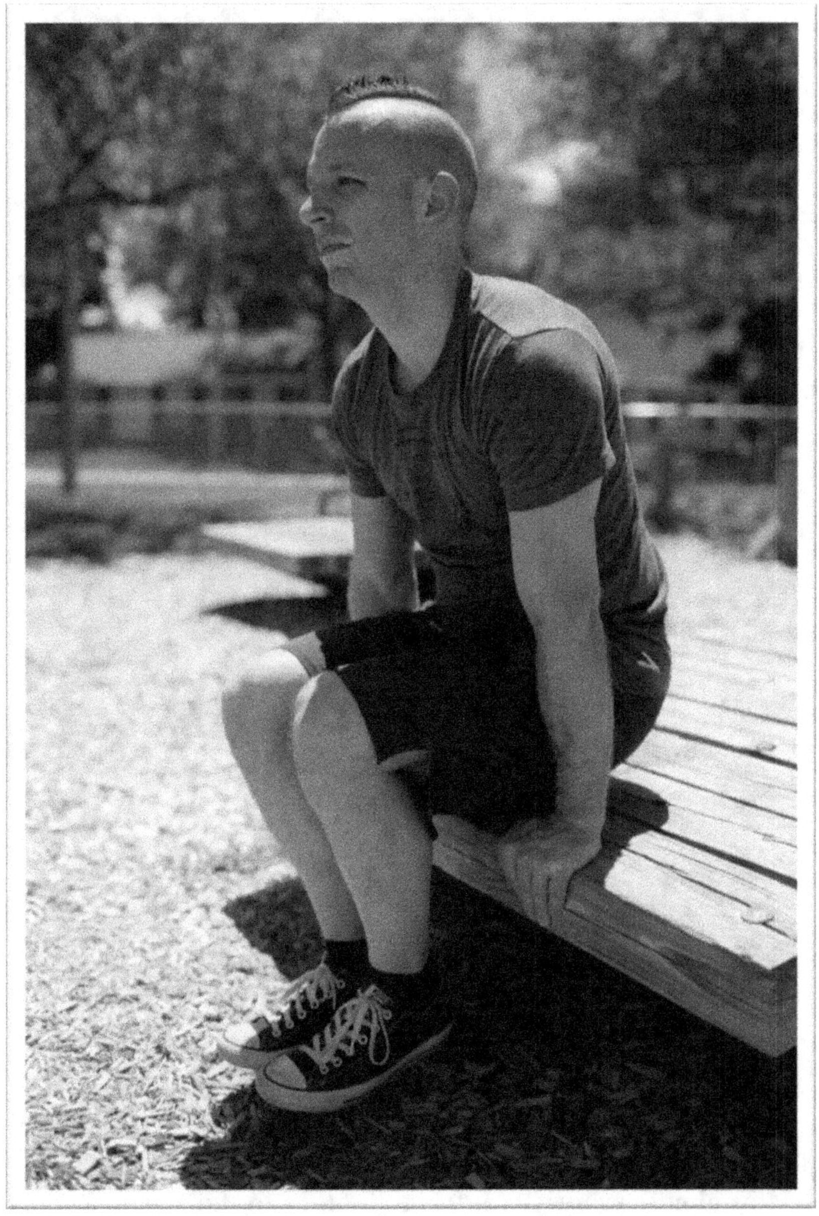

Bent Leg L-Sit, a.k.a. the N-Sit, is more of a hold position. Start with your hands on the ground or on a bench next to your butt. Lift your butt up off the ground with your knees tucked up towards your chest. If it is a struggle at first, then try it on an elevated surface.

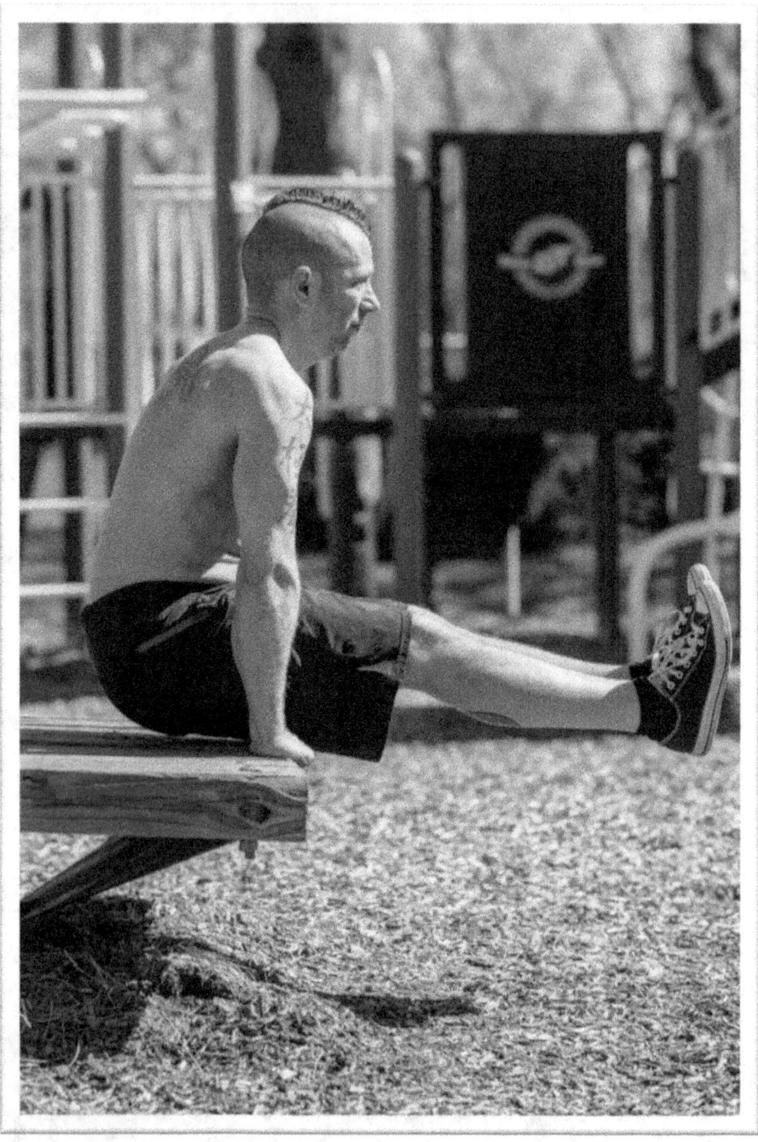

L-sits are a step up from the bent leg version. To be honest, I have done this almost everywhere, from an office to the sidewalk. Sitting on the floor or a bench, place your hands right next to your butt and lift yourself up and extend your legs straight out and hold it. This can also be done on parallel bars or any other raised surface. To be honest, if you can't get yourself off the ground a raised surface may be best to start.

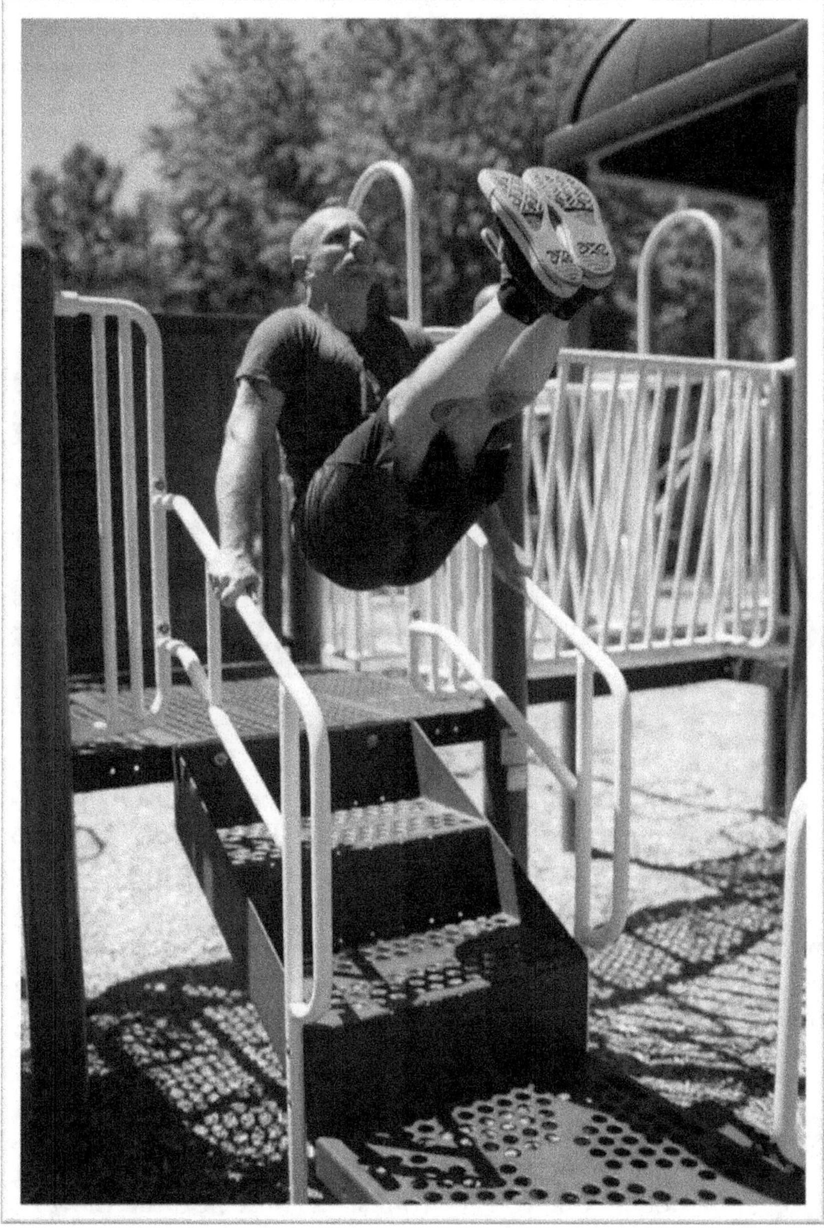

The V-Sit increases your range of motion on the L-Sit. Place your hands next to your butt and lift your butt up and extend your legs out. However, this time send them skyward. This will work the balance and the core, and up that burn to a new level.

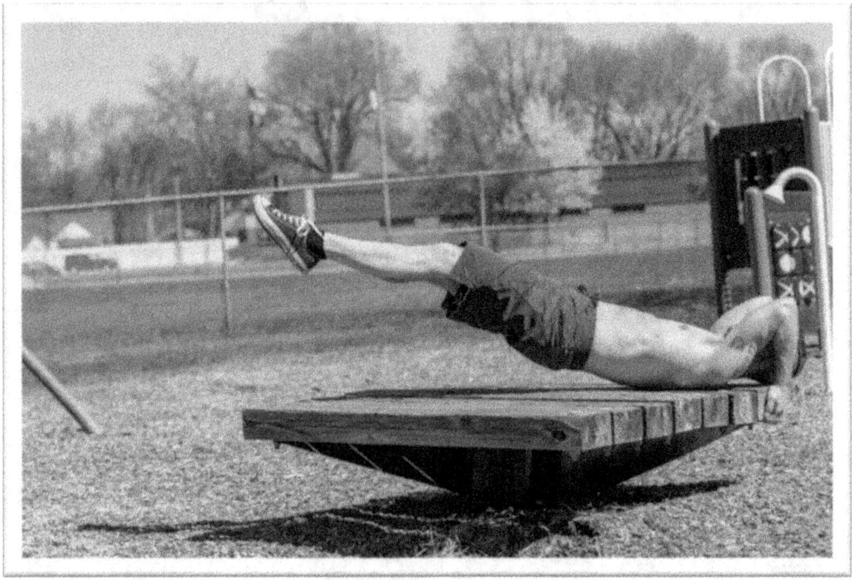

Dragon Flags are a beast worth conquering, but like many other things will take time. Start by lying on the ground, or a flat bench. You will need something to keep you anchored. From here tighten your core and lift your legs, hips and entire core straight up into a shoulder stand. Really work to nor pull on your neck. Once at the top, carefully lower yourself down holding your body as straight as possible until you are hovering just above the surface. Now, it is absolutely possible that you can't get there just yet, so here are some options to get you going. You can start by starting in a shoulder stand and lower yourself using negatives. You can also keep one knee tucked and lower down with just one leg extended.

You have worked on the ground and bench, so it is time to go to the bar. No, not the one you get drinks at. These next few moves will require a bit of grip strength, but they will pay off.

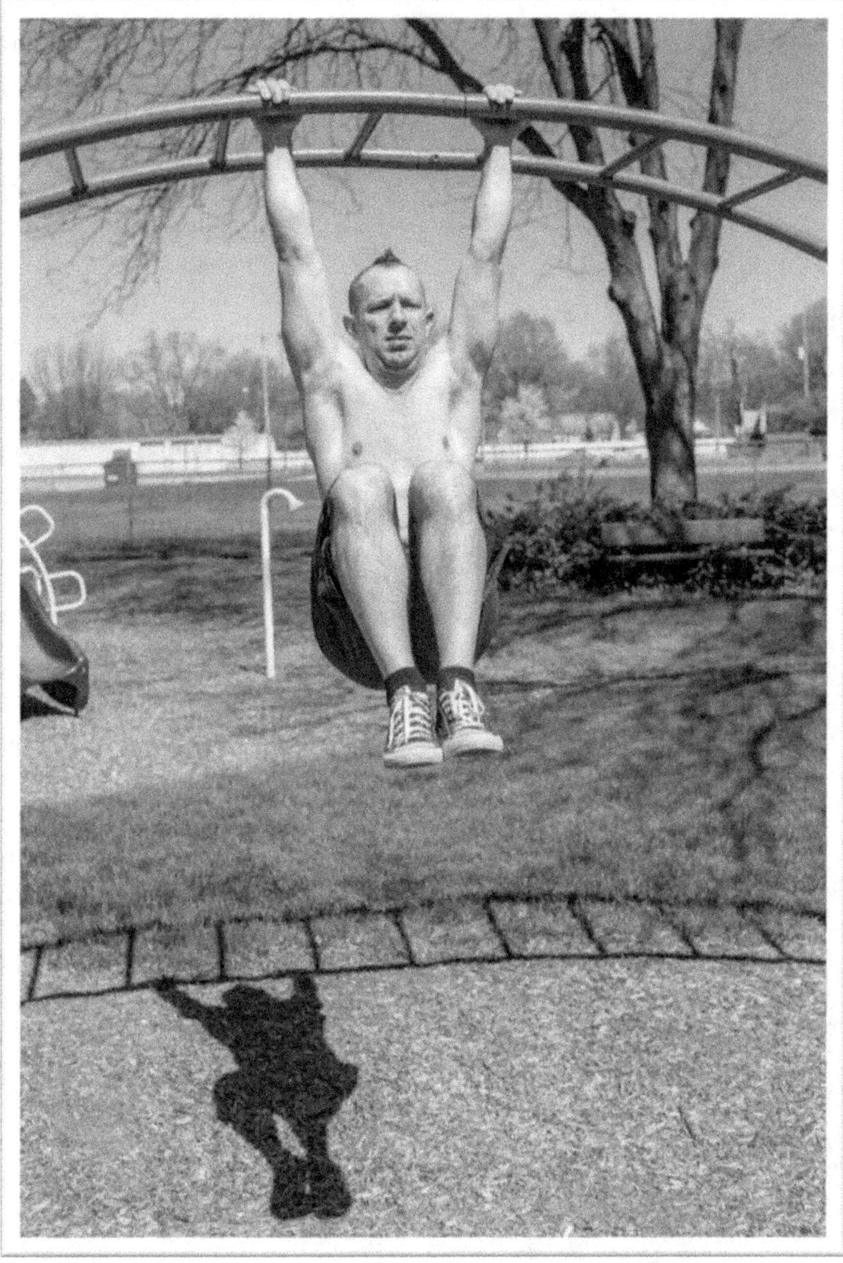

Hanging Knee Tucks start by hanging from the bar with arms straight. With legs extended and the core hollowed, carefully pull the knees up to the chest and lower them back down. Work your best to maintain control and prevent swinging on the bar.

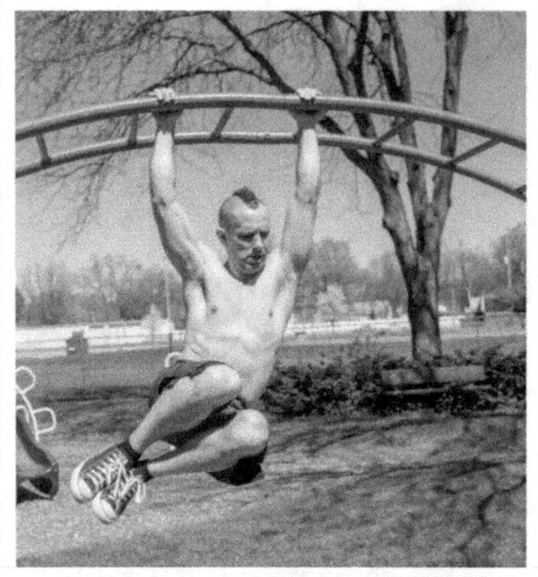

Twisting Hanging Knee Tucks start by hanging from the bar. Twist your core and pull your knees up to your opposite armpit. Lower your legs back down without swinging, then repeat on the other side. Fight to keep your arms straight throughout the movement.

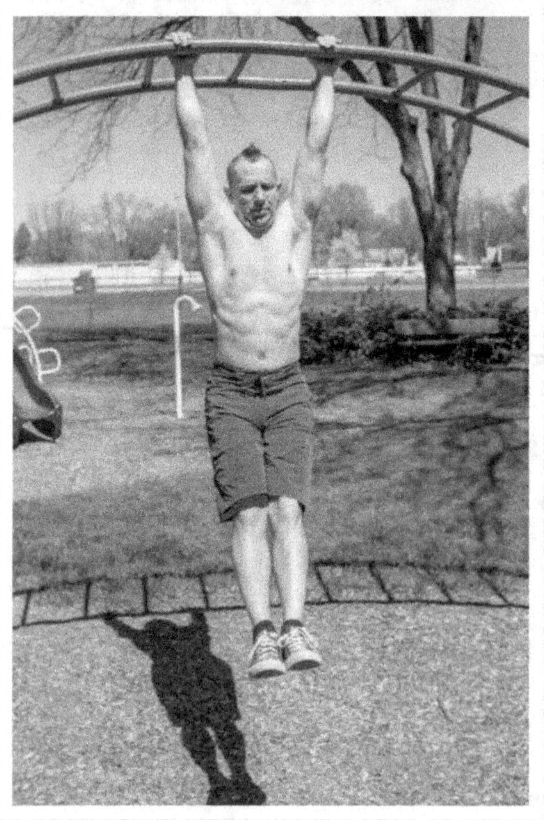

Straight Leg Raise starts with hanging from the bar like you are at the bottom of a pull-up. Fully engage your body and keeping straight legs bring your legs up to waist height and lower then back down. Try your best not to bend your arms, swing or use momentum to bring the legs up. This exercise is about control.

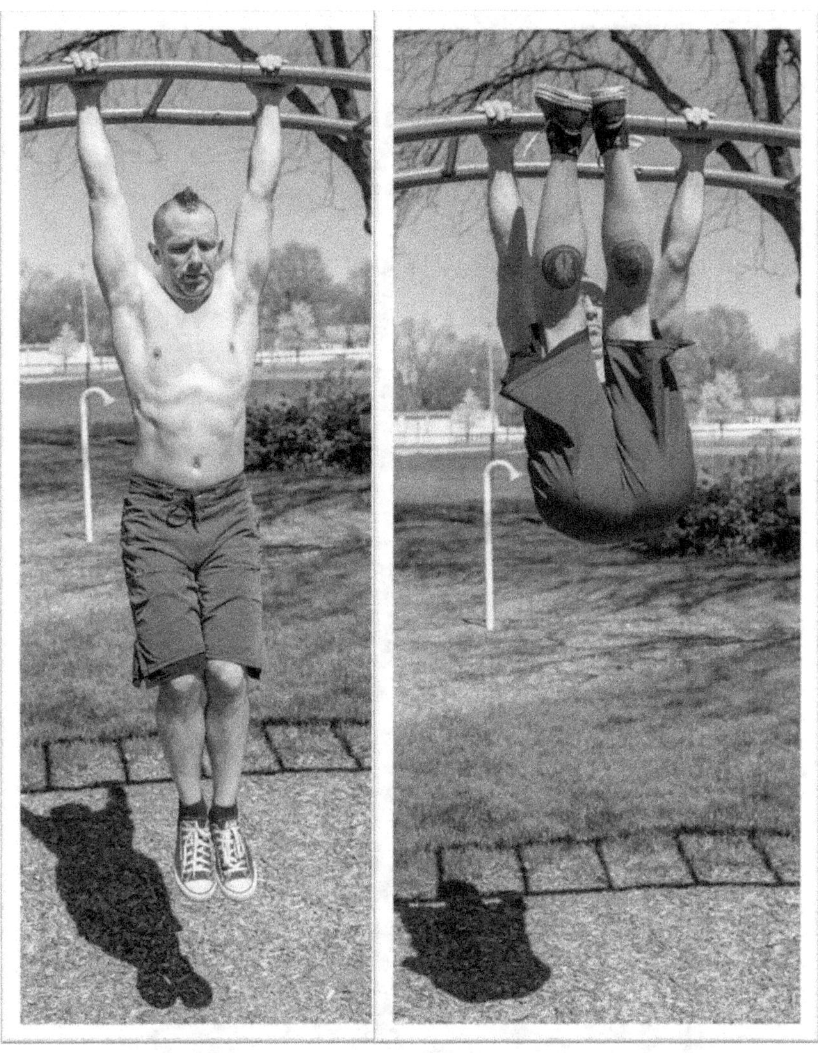

Toes to Bar Leg Raise is the next step up from the Straight Leg Raise. Hanging from the bar, engage your body and with straight legs bring your toes all the way up to tap the bar. With all the control you can muster, lower your straight legs back down. Once again, be careful not to swing. As you progress, this can also be done with just one arm.

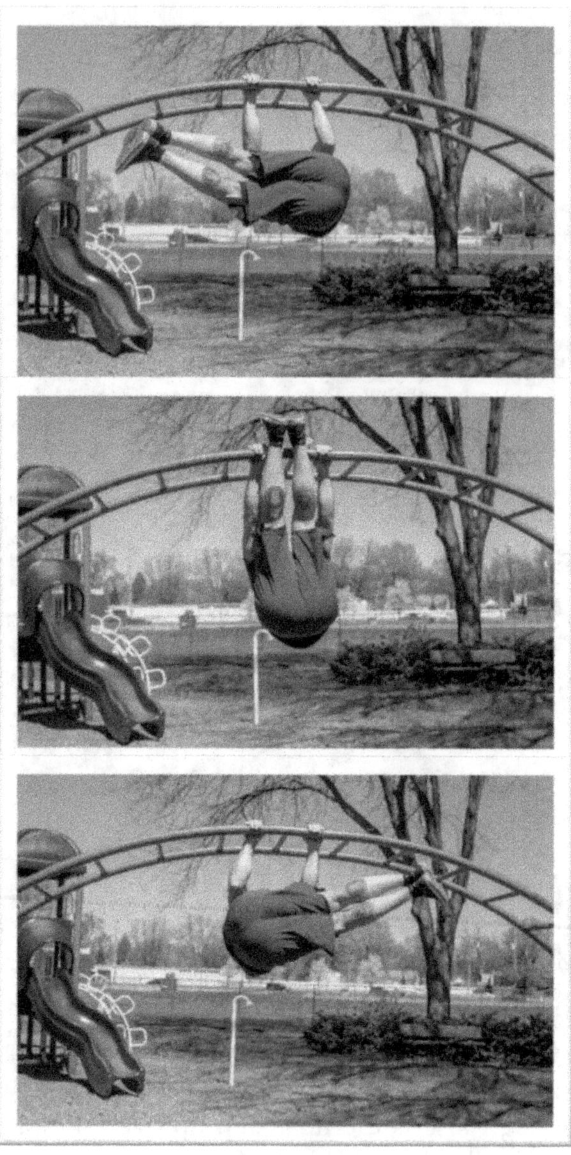

Windshield Wipers begin with bringing your toes all the way up to the bar with straight legs and arms. Once at the top, rotate your legs down to your side and repeat on the other side. This will take some serious muscle control as well as grip strength. At first keeping the legs and arms completely straight may be rough, but give it your best shot. It will get better with time.

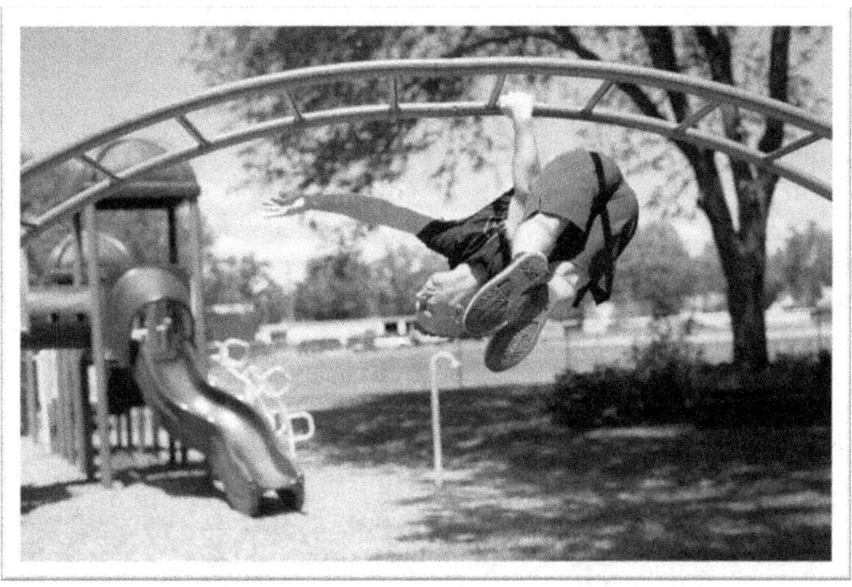

The Meat Hook was an exercise that took me a while to be able to do. So, don't worry if you don't get it right away. This will take a few progressions to get here, but I'm here to lay it out for you. The first thing you will need to nail down, is a one arm bar hang. You need grip strength on your side. Next I would suggest to have the windshield wipers down; this move takes a lot of core rotation. Let's start on your strong side. Start by pulling yourself up to windshield wiper position. Then, lower your legs all the way over to your strongest side. Now, roll your hips up towards your elbow almost folding around your arm. This will take a few tries to find that balance spot. Once you have it, slowly and carefully release one finger at a time on your weak side. Once you have released the hand try to hold it for a few seconds. Achievement Unlocked: Meat Hook! Remember to try to train both sides.

Chapter 14
Build Bridges Not Walls

So many people, including myself in the beginning, spend a lot of time slouching and not taking care of our backs. As we continue to do this the sitting slouch turns into a walking hunch, and that hunch can be one bad hombre. As a matter of fact, correcting this is one of the first things I do when I'm working with my martial art classes as well as my one-on-one clients. So now we look at the opposite position for the body, Bridging or Back Bends. I'm sure while you are reading this, many of you are thinking, "I'm not flexible enough to do that". Don't worry, like everything else it just requires some time and training. Now, these moves are not just for building that flexibility, they can also be performed to build strength in the lower back, shoulders, glutes and hamstrings. So in a way, this can be a good replacement for those deadlifts. The major obstacle at first may be your current flexibility. We will work on that.

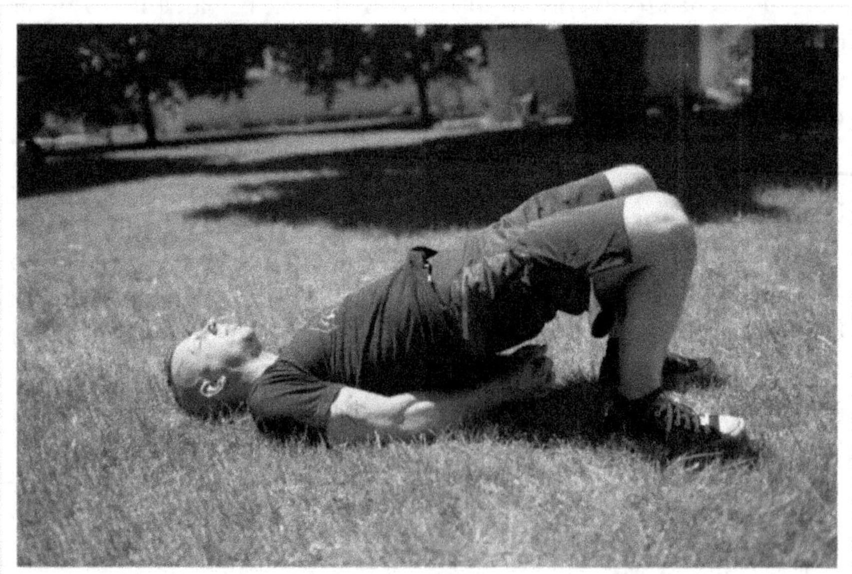

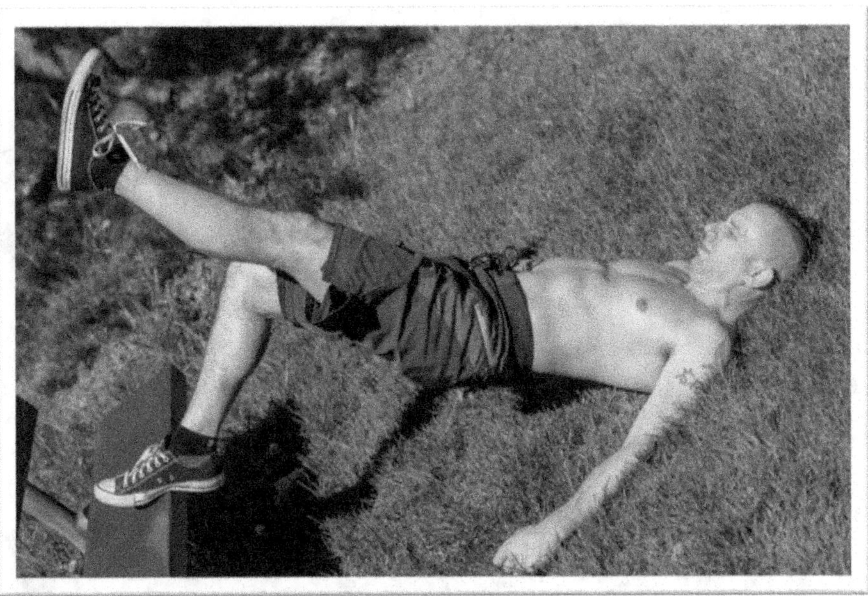

Hip Thrusters or Hip Bridges are great! But looks kinda dirty... Yeah... So, there are a few ways to do this. The easiest way is to put your back on a bench and with feet planted on the ground about knee distance from you, push your hips to the sky until you are as level as a table. To increase the challenge, move off the bench and onto the ground. Next, try to move the shoulder blades together and interlace your fingers behind your back. If you do it for reps, then keep the hands on the ground. Once that gets kinda easy, try elevating your feet or do it with just one leg on the ground or bench. This will for sure work the booty and hamstrings.

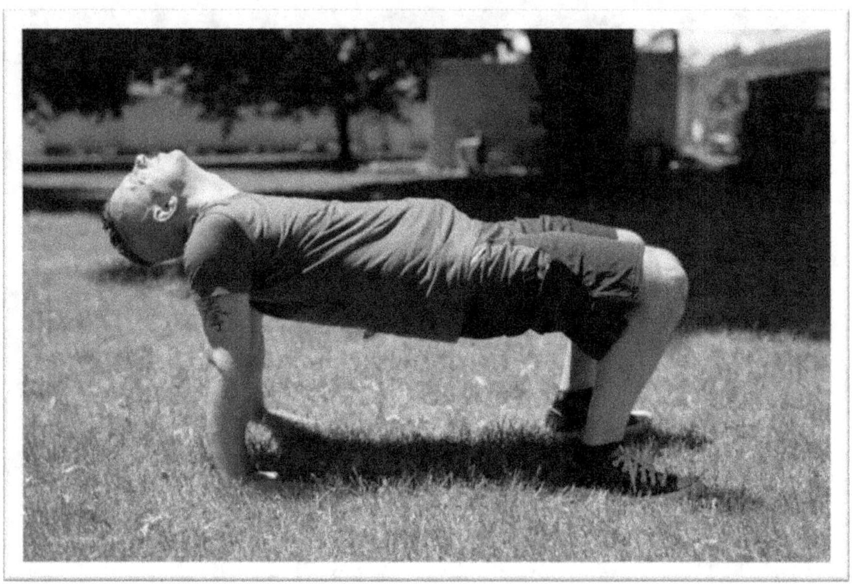

Table Bridge transform! Sitting on the ground with your feet flat and palms on the ground. You can toy around with having your fingers pointed in or out. From here press your hips up flattening out your body to a table. Press your chest out and open up the shoulders. You can also drop your head back.

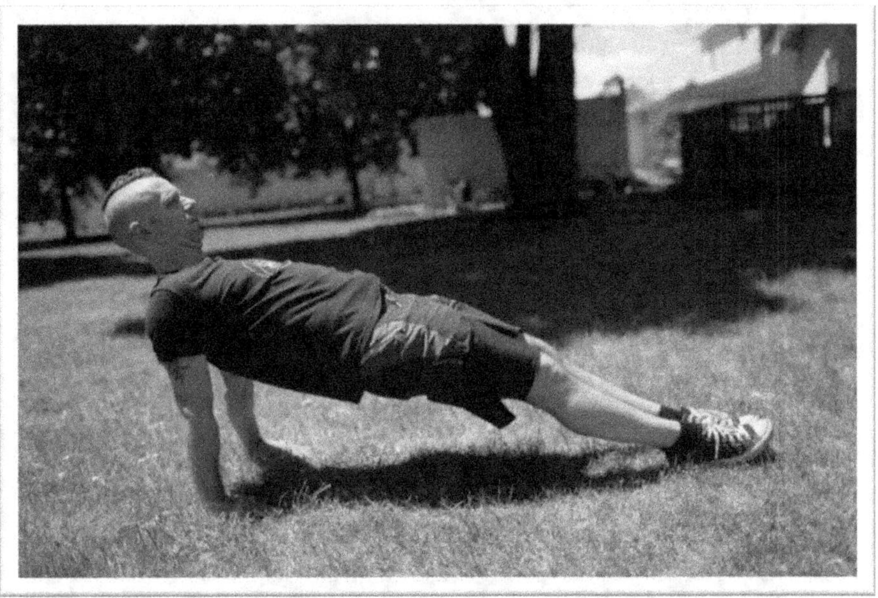

The Straight Bridge starts out sitting on the ground with your legs straight out. Place the hands flat on the ground, again you can play around with the hand position a bit. Lift yourself up and flatten out our body, keeping only your hands and heels on the ground. Drop your head back and try to engage your entire core to keep the body straight. This can also be done with just one leg to increase the difficulty. If you do this, then remember to work both sides to keep it even.

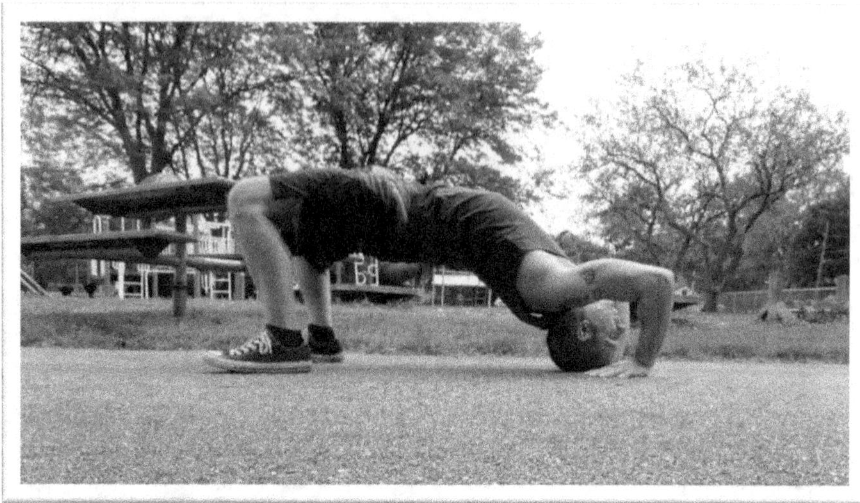

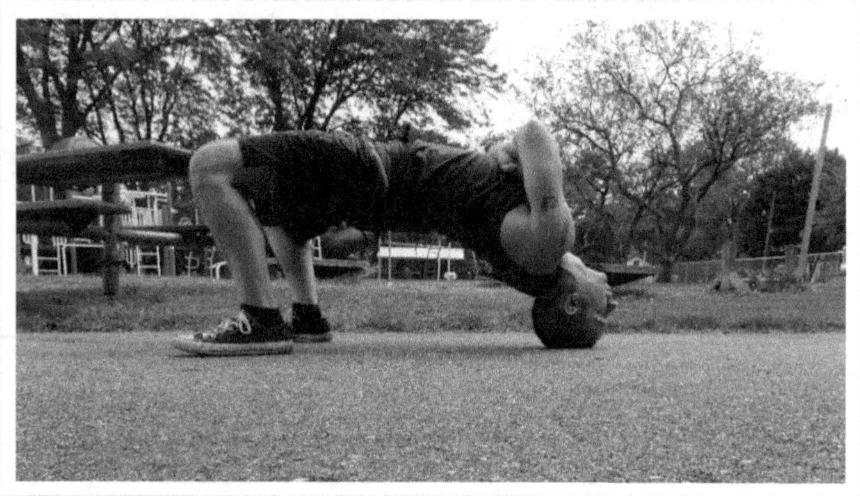

Head Bridges not only work the entire posterior chain, but work the neck, too. To start, lay on your back on the floor... not to nap... Bend your knees and plant your feet on the ground. For your first time doing this, plant your hands palms down with fingers pointing towards the shoulders. Do this while, pressing your chest into the air and arch your spine, roll up on the palms and the top of your head. As you get comfortable in this position, you can remove your hands from the ground and just balance on your head.

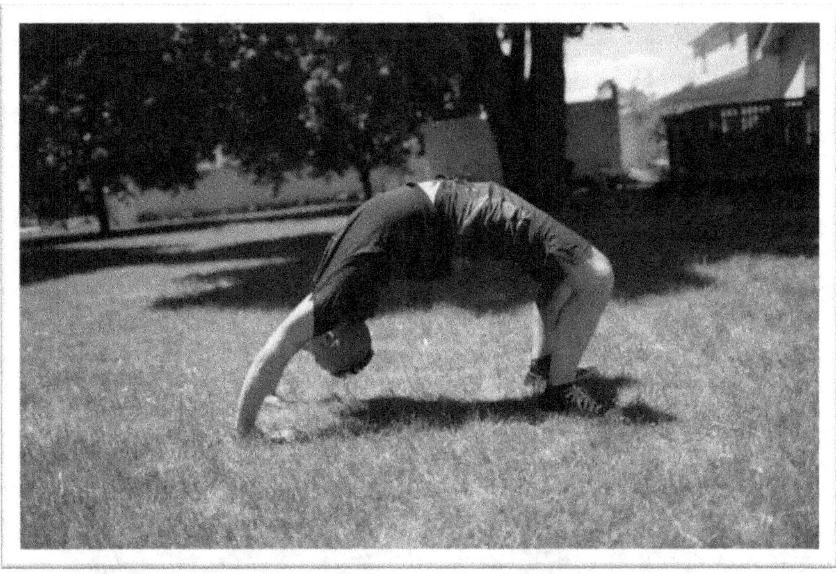

Back Bridges can be a little too much for some people's spines. But, with a bit of work you can cross this bridge. Get down on the ground on your back to get started. Bend your knees bringing your feet close to your butt. Place the hands flat on the ground next to your head with fingers pointed towards your shoulders. From here push your chest and abs up to the sky extending your arms out as far as you can arching your spine. At first you may not be able to get your arms completely locked out. Now, your back may not be super arched just yet, but keep training it and it will get better. Another way I have trained for this is walking down the wall with my hands, like a certain friendly neighborhood wall crawler we all know and love. Walk your hands as far down as you can. There is a chance your hands will not make it to the floor on the first several tries. Like the other bridges, when you are comfortable you can switch to single leg.

Chapter 15
Flying with Plyometrics!

Some heroes have jumps and some just straight up fly. This section is to get you off the ground to new heights in new ways. Before you really jump into this, make sure you have the basic movements down first. Don't feel you have to go into this before you are ready. It will again take time and will put a lot of extra stress on your joints if you don't prepare them. No super hero landings, despite the other heroes doing it. It is totally impractical and bad on your knees.

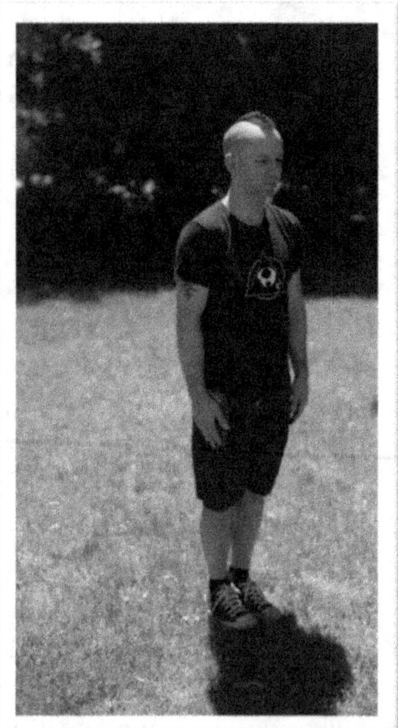
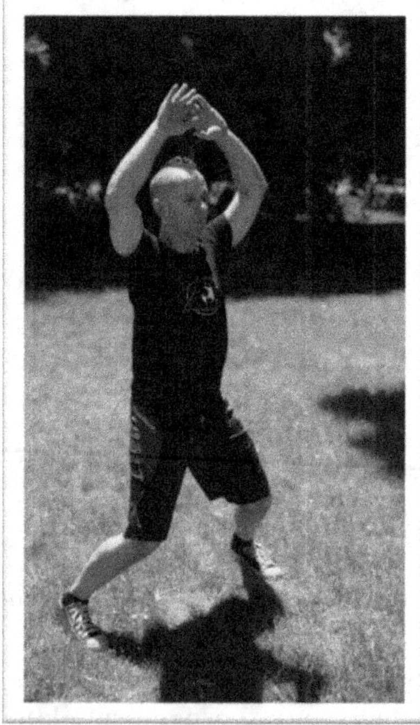

Jumping Jacks are probably one of the best known plyo exercises. Start by standing tall, with feet together and arms at your side. From here jump your feet apart and swing your arms up above your head. Then back to starting position. This can be a great way to warm up your entire body.

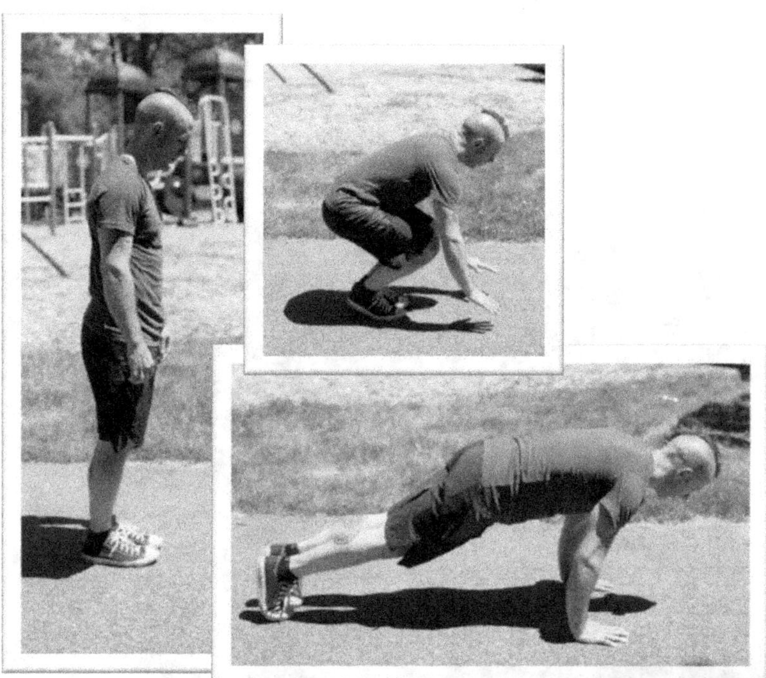

The Infamous Burpee! Most have seen them, and most don't like them. I love them. Stand tall like the hero you are, and extend your arms up over head. Simultaneously squat down and place your hands on the ground. From here shoot your legs out into a high plank. Jump them back in, and from the squat jump up into the air. When coming back down land soft and repeat.

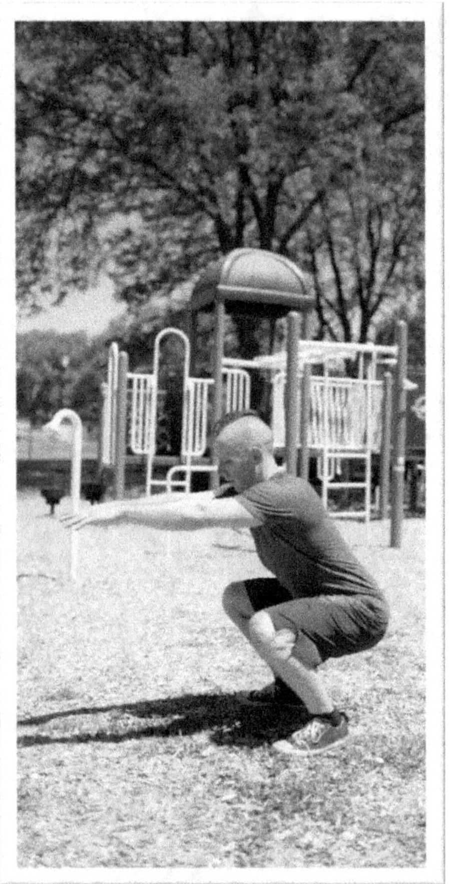 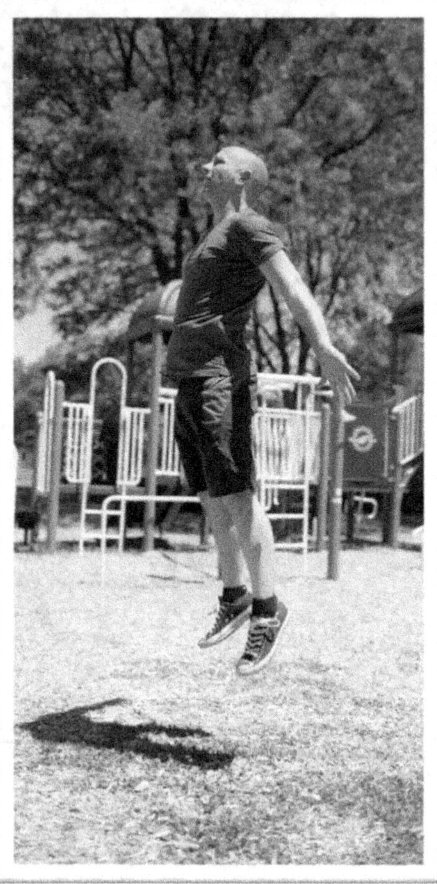

Squat Jumps is your first trip into the sky. Sink your body down into a deep squat, once at the bottom push yourself up as fast and hard as you can to leave the ground. When you land you want to land with soft knees and toes first, rolling down to your heels.

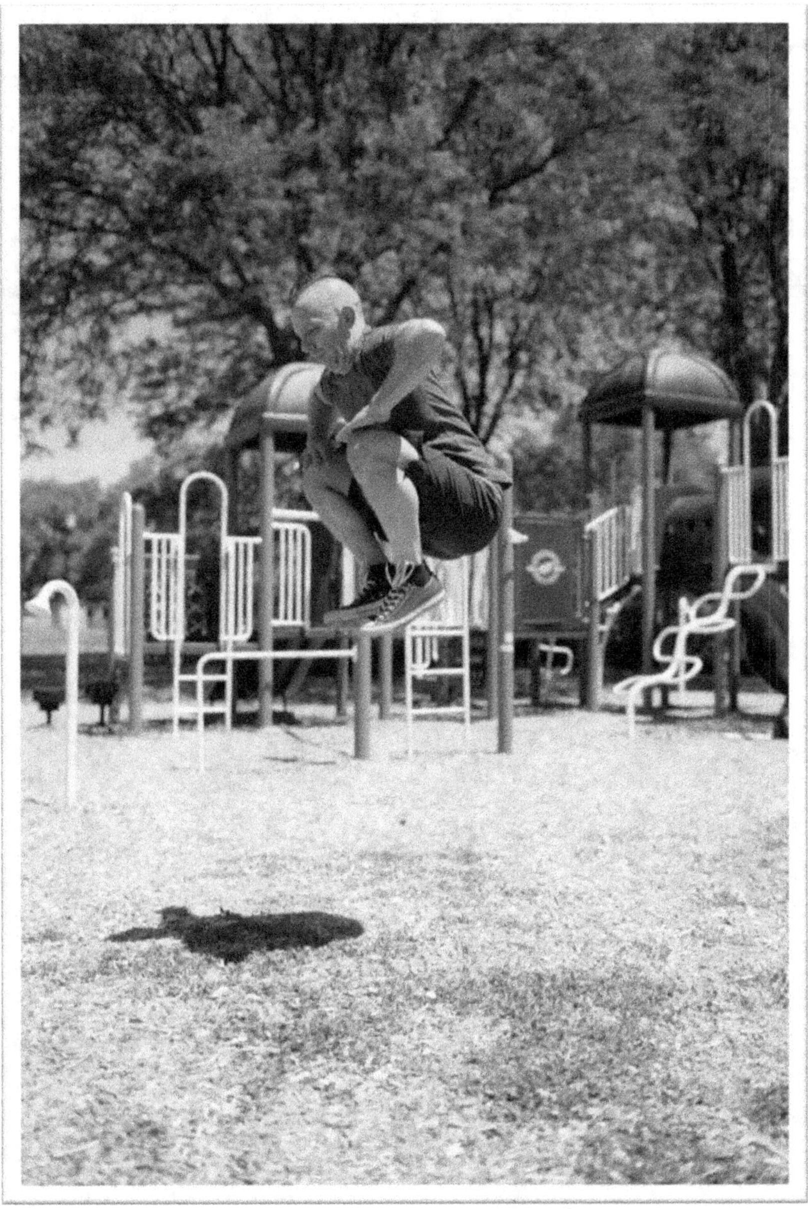

Tuck Jumps use a high jump not necessarily implementing a squat. Power off the ground and while in the air tuck your knees to your chest. Again, land softly toes first rolling down to your heels. When you hit the ground try to make as little sound as possible. Land like a ninja.

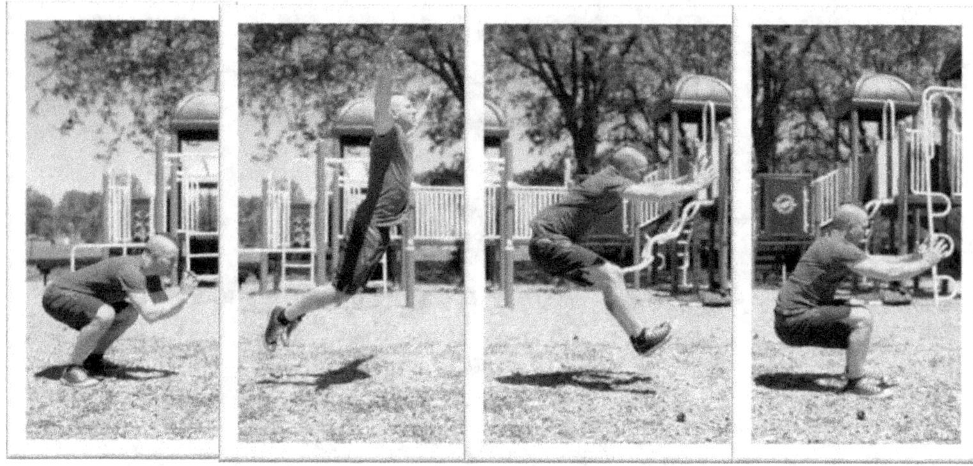

Long jumps are those old friends from the track and field days... Or the days you have to chase a super villain across roof tops. Start in that deep squat and push off hard with your feet propelling yourself forward as far as you can. In this jump you will have to land heels first but keep the knees soft.

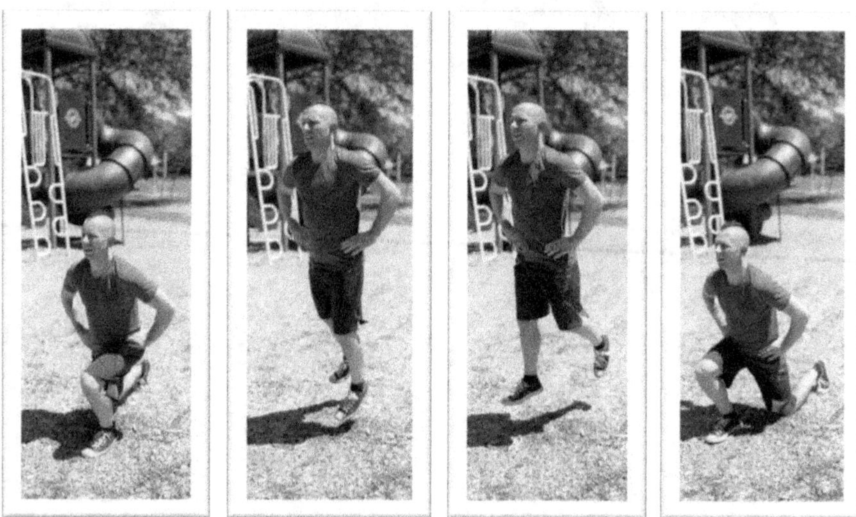

Split Jumps are great for building speed and power. Start off in a deep split squat or lunge. Explode up and switch feet in the air moving the front foot to the back and the back to the front. Most of the push should be coming from the front leg.

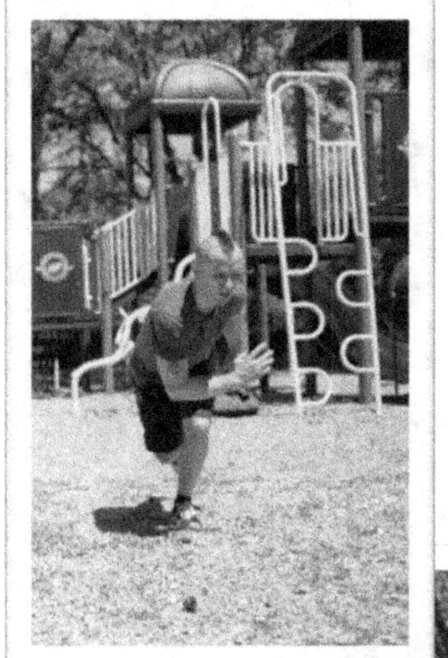

Speed Skater Jumps utilize a more side to side movement and a lot of power from one leg at a time. Standing on one foot, sink down as if you are doing a single leg squat letting the free leg just float out behind you. Once down, spring up pushing yourself towards the free leg. As you come

down switch to the other leg. Repeat on both sides. Remember to land as softly as possible.

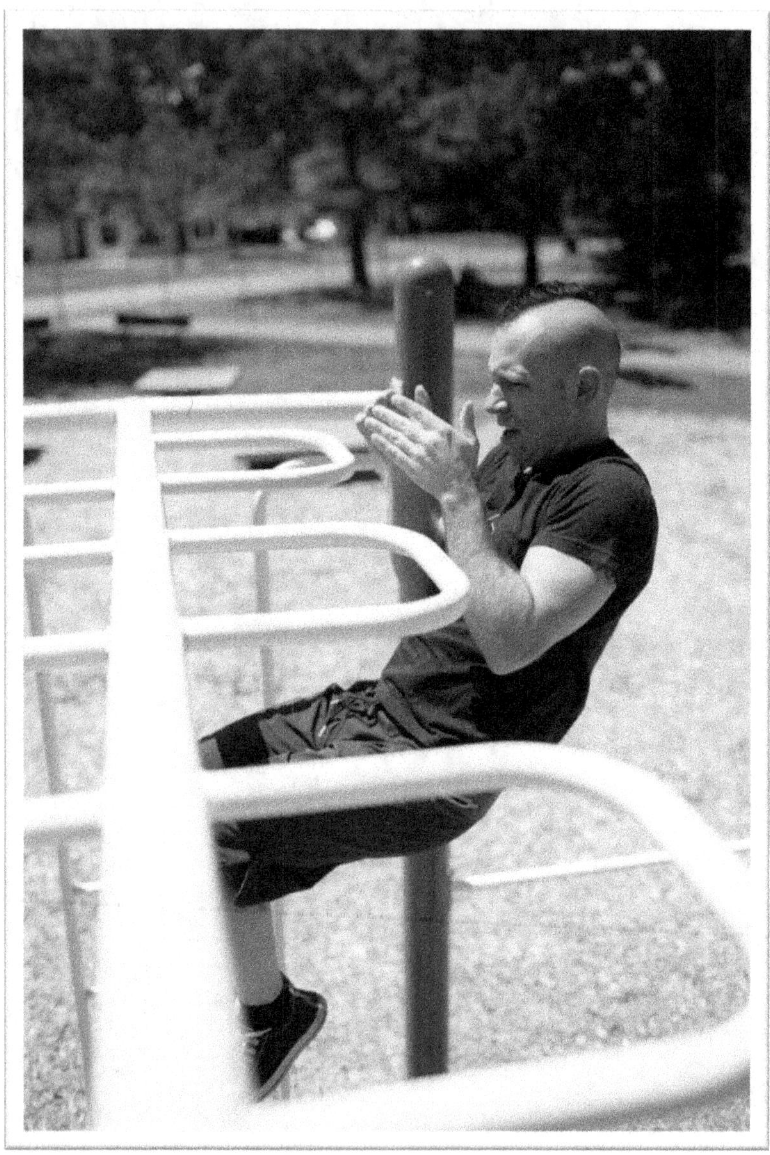

Plyometric Pull-Up is a tricky one. Sure, you can do a pull-up. But can you do it with such power that your hands can leave the bar? No, you don't have to clap, you just have to get off the bar. Start at the bottom of your pull up. Pull yourself up as fast as you can and release the bar, even if it is only a moment. Then, grab the bar and lower yourself back down.

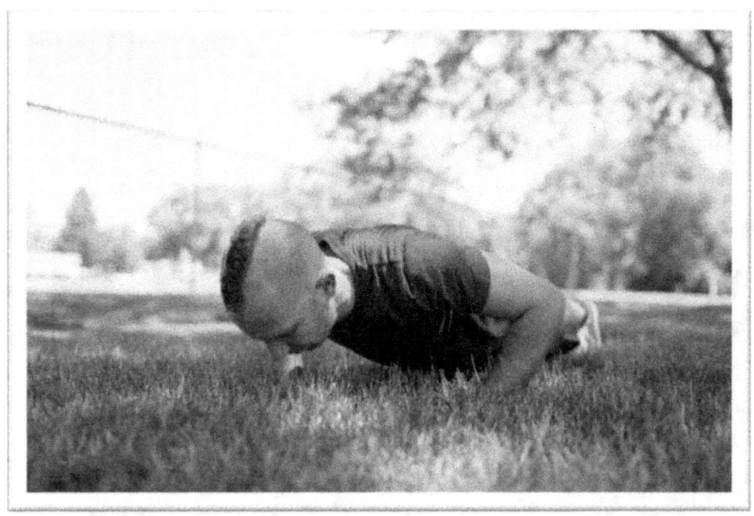

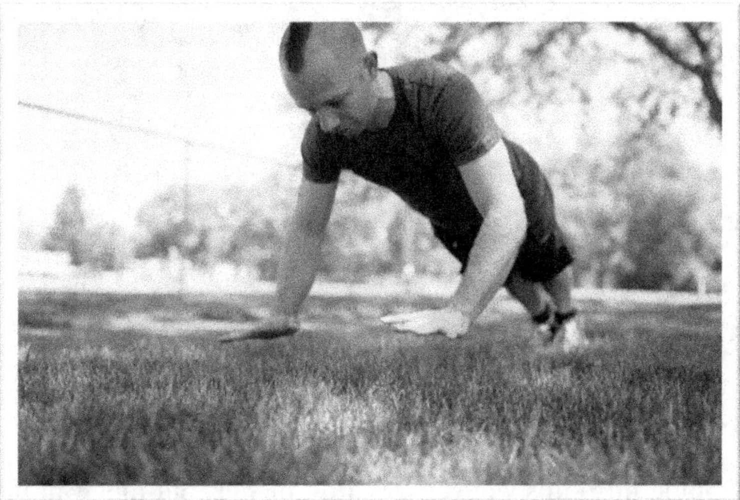

Pop Up Push-Up is going to be your first plyo push-up. Get into your classic push up position, lower yourself down and then push-up fast and hard to get your hands to just leave the ground. When landing keep the elbows relaxed to brace yourself on your return to earth.

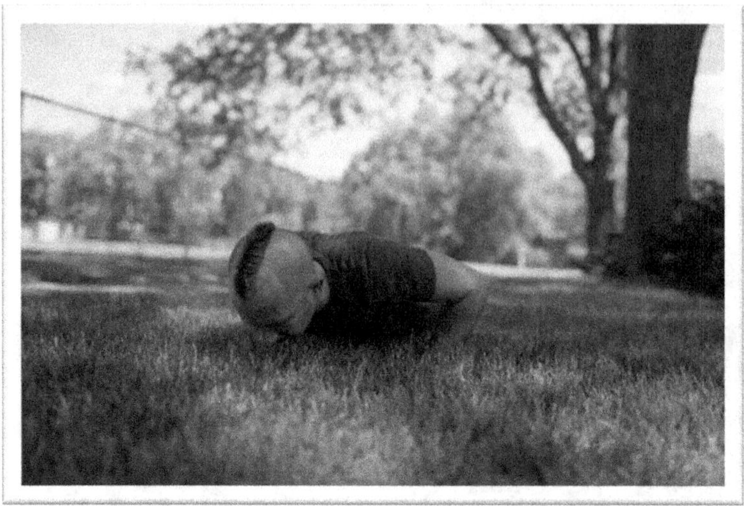

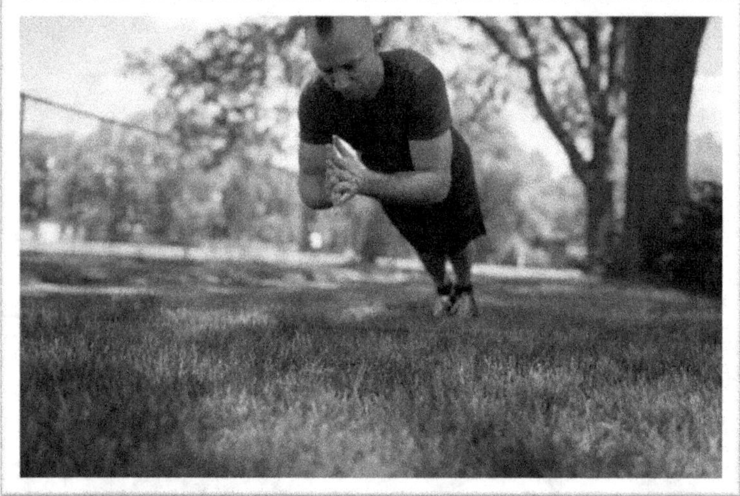

Clapping push-ups will get you a bit higher, but they will have to just to prevent that dreaded face plant. Again, get in that push-up position and lower yourself down. Then push the earth away from you as hard as you can. Once in the air, clap the hands, (even if it is just one quick clap) and on the way down catch yourself with hands back on the ground and keep the elbows soft. For an added challenge try getting the entire body off the ground. Give it maximum effort.

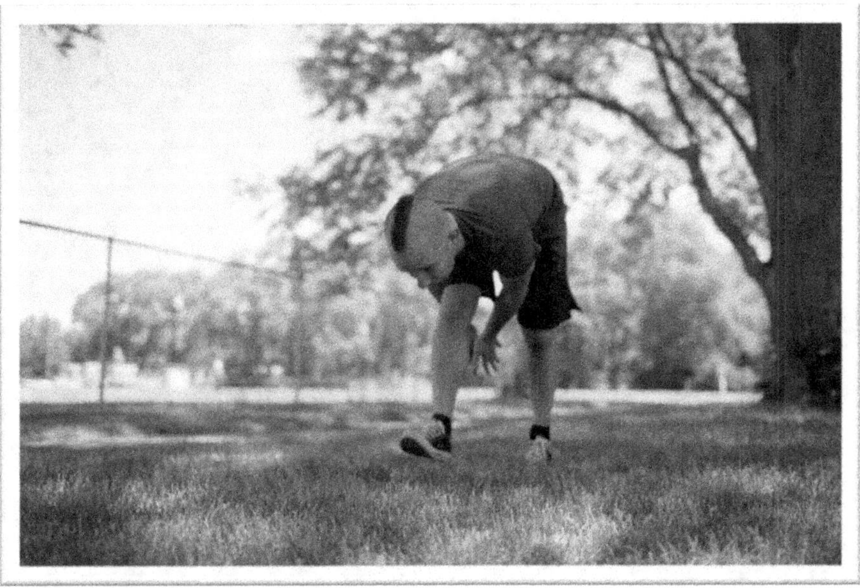

Behind the Knee Clapping Push-ups are at the very least tricky. You will need crazy speed, power and coordination. Get into your push-up position, lower yourself down and power off the ground. Once off the ground bring one knee forward towards your chest and clap behind it. Send the leg back, and work to land softly on your hands. You will have to be able to push yourself really high up to pull this off. When ready try it on both sides.

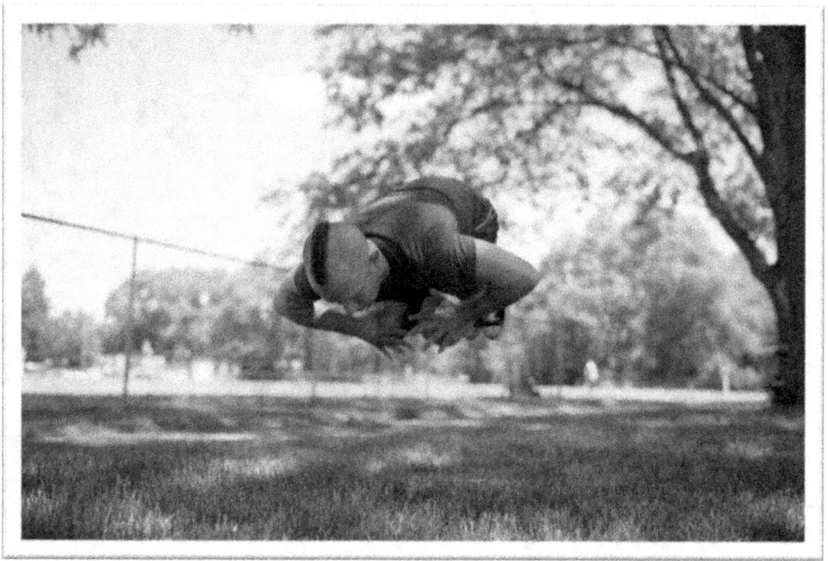

Knee Tap Push-ups take you fully off the ground again. Getting into that push-up, lower yourself down and push your entire body away from the earth. Once airborne tuck both knees into your chest and tap your knees with both hands. Now extend your body back out and catch yourself in push-up position. Again, this is a rather advanced move and will take some time. Don't rush to face this challenge.

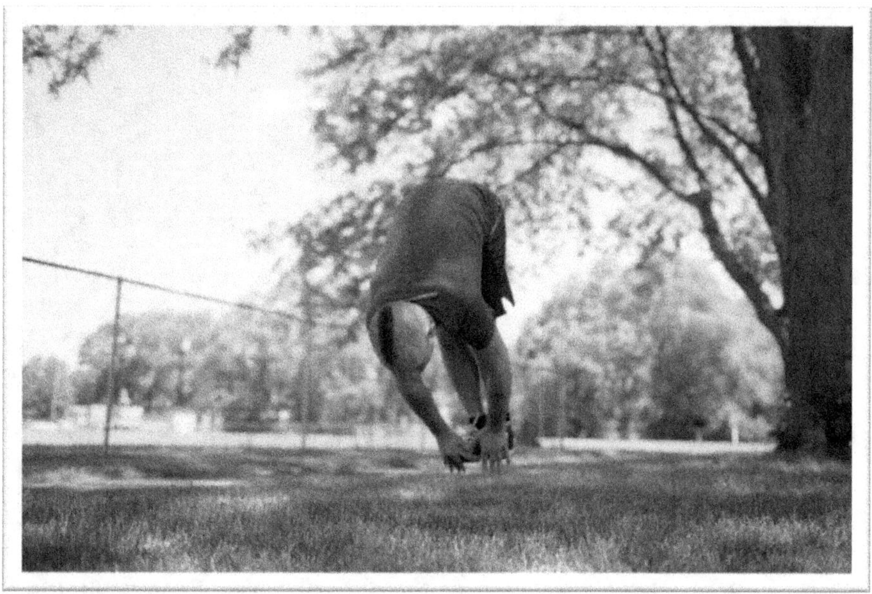

Aztec Push-Ups are no easy villain to face. This will fully test your speed and power. You need to get way high up to pull this off. As always, start off in your push-up. When yourself up to the sky you must pike in the air making almost an upside-down V. When here you need to tap your toes in mid-air. Then flatten back out to that push-up position. Unless you have a crazy healing factor, don't smash your face!

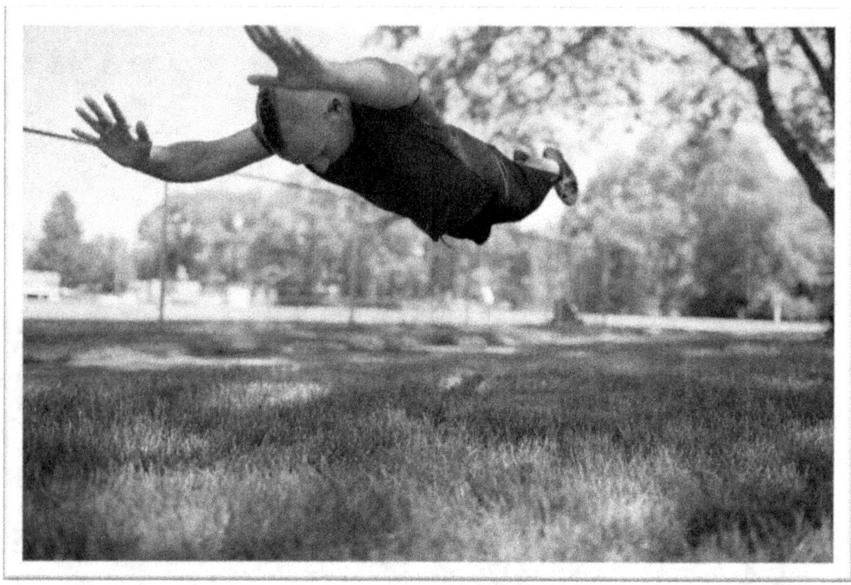

It's a Bird... It's a plane... No! It's the Superman Push-Up! This is super human flight! In this issue, you will need to push-up off the ground with everything your body can muster. When your entire body is up in the sky, reach your arms out overhead like the man of steel himself. As you return to earth, catch yourself softly in push-up position.

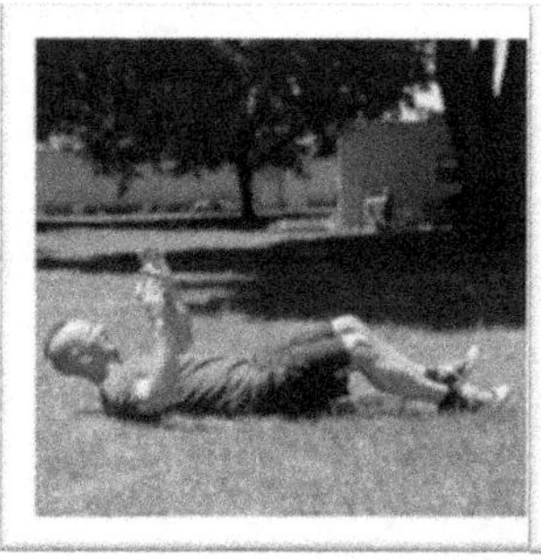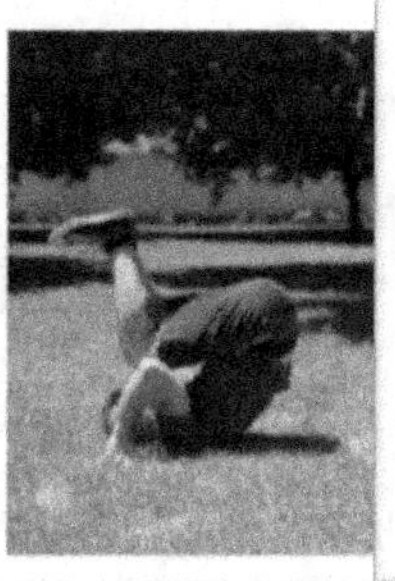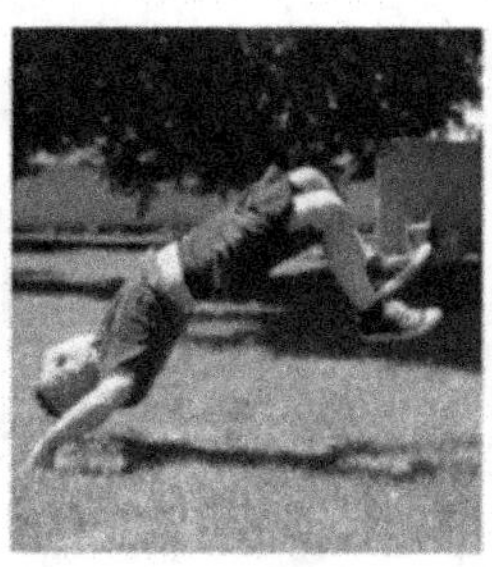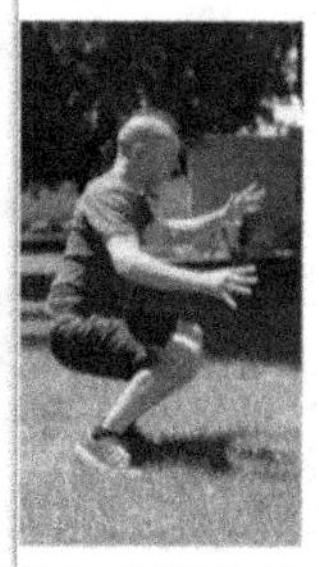

The Kip-Up is the ultimate Ninja/Kung Fu move. We have seen it in movies and TV shows. The hero gets knocked to the floor and gets ups with a jump from his back to his feet! To be honest, this will take a lot of tries to get it down and at first you may look like a flopping fish on dry land. With the back arch that you will use to perform this, it is really like a moving bridge. Start off laying on your back on the ground and place your hands flat on the ground next to your head. Tuck your knees in towards your chest and start rolling towards your shoulders. Kick your legs up with all your super strength and push off with your hands. Everything explodes up while in the air you create a arch in the back as you land on your feet ready to continue the fight. This move will take power and precision timing.

Final thoughts:

This is your journey, so enjoy it. No two people will progress the same, nor does anyone have the exact same build, so focus on you. I know if you want it bad enough you will achieve great things. Quest Fitness is always here to help you out when you have questions or concerns. Even though this is designed as an 8 week program, take your time on your quest and listen to your body. Some months may need to be extended an extra week, and that's ok. As I said before, this is not a complete guide to calisthenics. Once you have the basics, expand your knowledge. You are capable of unlimited potential. The most important thing I can say in closing is, do this for YOU and no one else.

Chapter 16
The Quest Begins

Here is where it starts. All the exercises listed are suggestions to get you started. But all the exercises can be progressed and regressed based on your current level. So, if you can't quite do a push-up or pull-up, then use the info from earlier in the book to get started. As you progress you can change it up, but try to stick to the system in place. This is how you will conquer your fitness goals.

Character Building:

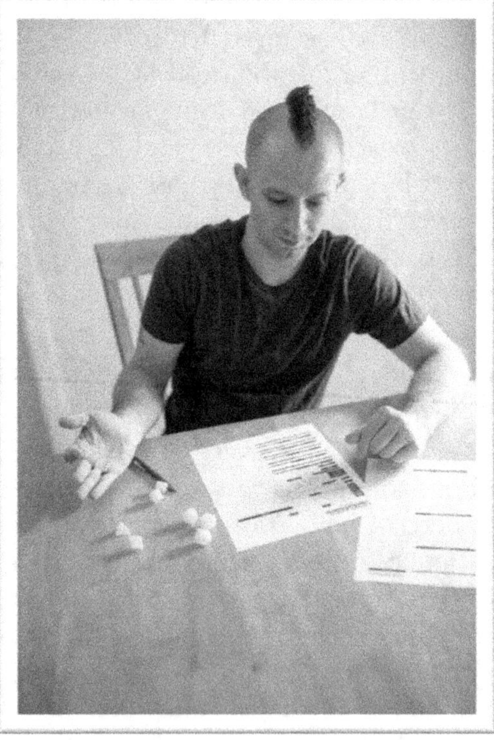

This is your start, where you rollout the foundation of your calisthenics journey, and where you will first face your greatest rival, yourself. It is recommended that everyone start here. It also isn't a bad idea to revisit this from time to time to prevent that dreaded plateau. In this section you need to focus on form and quality of movement over number of reps. You will notice the most rest days in the first month, this is to ease you into your workout if it is your first workout in a long time. On the non-workout days, you should be on the active rest the was discussed before. Again, you can stay in this phase rotating between month 1 & 2 for as long as you need, before you move on. Remember this is your fitness journey.

Month One: Week 1-4

Day 1 & 5: On these days the suggested set number is 2-3 with rep range is 8-12, and 30 second rest between sets. So, your first 2-3 sets will be push-ups immediately followed by pull-ups then a 30 second rest then repeat. Keep in mind all the exercises are the recommended versions, but they can be progressed and regressed based on your current fitness level. In this phase you will be using a movement tempo of 3/2/1. What does this mean? Well, you will lower yourself down using a 3 second count, 2 second hold under tension, then a 1 second movement back to the tensions position.

Exercise

| Push-Up |
| Pull-up |
| |
| Squats |
| Single leg deadlifts |
| |
| Bench Dips |
| Chin ups |
| |
| Hip Thrusters |
| Split squats |

Day 3: This is your cardio day! This will be done through Tabata training. What is Tabata you ask? It is 20 seconds giving it your all followed by a 10 seconds rest. Each exercise is 4-6 rounds. Sure, 20 seconds doesn't seem like much, but give it a try then we can talk.

Jumping jacks
Burpees
Push up shoulder tap.
Squat jumps
Mountain climbers
Side to side plank walk
Sitting knee tucks
High plank to low plank

Core: This is a great start to start your core training. Each one of these exercises should be performed for 30 seconds each for 2-3 sets with a 30 second rest. The core can be trained up to 3 days a week. I would suggest adding it in right after the other workouts.

Plank
Side plank
Floor cobra

Month 2: Week 5-9

Day 1, 3 & 5: On these days the suggested set number is 2-3 with rep range is 8-12, immediately after you finish the reps, you hold a movement under tension for up to 30 seconds then take 30 to 60 second rest between sets. Keep in mind all the exercises are the recommended versions, but they can be progressed and regressed based on your current fitness level. In this phase you will be using a movement tempo of 3/2/1. What does this mean? Well, you will lower yourself down using a 3 second count, 2 second hold under tension, then a 1 second movement back to the tensions position.

Push-ups / ISO push-up
Pull up / iso pull
Bench dips / dip hold
Chin up / iso hold
Squats / wall sits
Single leg deadlifts / shoulder bridge
Lunges / iso hold
Hip thrusters / iso hold shoulder bridge

Day 2: This is your cardio day! This will be done through Tabata training. What is Tabata you ask? It is 20 seconds giving it your all followed by a 10 seconds rest. Each exercise is 4-6 rounds. Sure, 20 seconds doesn't seem like much, but give it a try then we can talk.

Jumping jacks
Burpees
Push up shoulder tap.
Squat jumps
Mountain climbers
Side to side plank walk
Sitting knee tucks
High plank to low plank

Pick Your Path:

Each one of the next 3 paths have different advantages, but all will get you fit. Read through them and find what you think will suit you best. Don't worry, you can always go back and try another path later. You are welcome to add in the following Ab workouts to each program. I would recommend doing abs 1-3 days a week after your scheduled workout if you choose to add them.

Ab routine 1

Do each move back to back for 2-3 sets with a 30 second rest at the end of each circuit.

Mountain Climbers 30 seconds
Laying Leg Lift 12 reps
Plank Toe tap 30 Seconds
Sitting Knee Tucks 12 reps
L-sit or V-sit 30 Seconds

Ab routine 2

Do each move back to back for 2-3 sets with a 30 second rest at the end of each circuit.

Hanging Leg Raise 12 Reps
Slow Mountain Climbers (Per Leg) 12 Reps
Hanging Twisting Knee Tucks (Per Side) 12 reps
Flutter Kicks (Per Leg) 12 Reps
Tuck And Crunch 12 Reps

The Powerhouse:

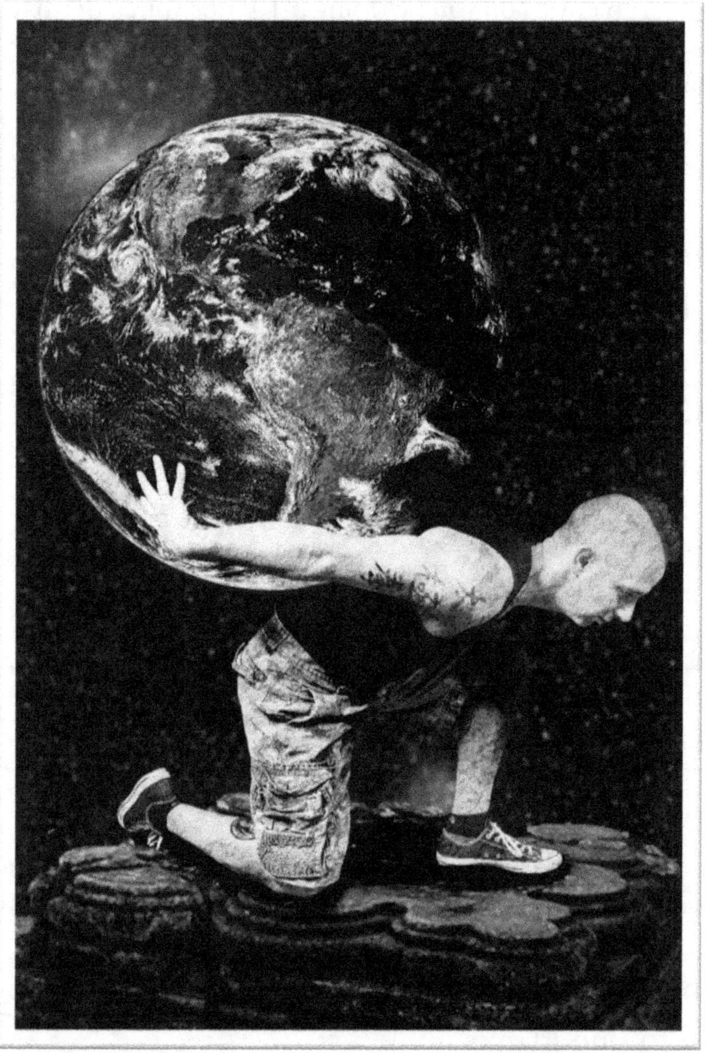

SMASH! This program is simplistic, basic and built for raw strength. Sure, there may be a few skills to pick up along the way, but this path is all about strength. The movements will be slow, and the range of your motions will be deep. But the reps will be lower in most cases. Through this program you are welcome to train a few of the stunts listed earlier in the book, just don't forget raw strength is the goal.

Month 1:

On the rep days You will be doing 8-10 reps with a 3/1/3 tempo at 3-4 sets. There will be a few exceptions where you will just hold a move under tension.

Day 1:

Pull-Up
Archer Pull-up
Front Lever Swing
Chin-Up
Hanging L-Sit Hold (15-30 Seconds)

Day 2:

Push-up
Archer Push-Up
Parallel Bar Dip
Decline Push-up
Straight Bar Dip

Day 3:

Cardio day! Each move is 30 seconds done back to back with a 1 min rest at the end of the circuit. Repeat the circuit 3-4 times.

Jumping Jacks
Side to side Planks
Knee Tucks
Speed Skater
Burpee
Bear Crawl
Squat Jump

Day 4:

Split Squat
Pistol Squat
Single Leg Hip Thruster
Archer Squat
Single Leg Dead Lift
Wall Sit (60 Seconds)

Day 5:

Angle Flag (Hold as long as possible)
Reverse Grip Rows
Pike Press
Planche Push-Up
Skin the Cat
Crow Pose (Hold As long as possible)

Month 2:

In this Super Human Strength month the tempo changes to 2/1/2, but the reps change with each set! Welcome to pyramids! You will climb up and down the pyramid. What is this craziness?!? Well if you see 8/10/12 after a exercise, it means set 1 is 8 reps, set 2 is 10, set 3 is 12reps, set 4 is 10 reps, set 5 is 8 reps. After each set you take a 30 second rest.

Day 1:

Pull-Up	6/8/10
Chin-Up	6/8/10
Front Lever (This is a hold)	5/7/9
One Arm Rows	6/8/10

Day 2:

One Arm Push-Up (per arm)	6/8/10
Straight Bar Dip	6/8/10
Decline Push-Up	6/8/10
Skull Crusher	6/8/10

Day 3:

Cardio day! Each move is 30 seconds done back to back with a 1 min rest at the end of the circuit. Repeat the circuit 3-4 times.

Jumping Jacks
Side to side Planks
Knee Tucks
Speed Skater
Burpee
Bear Crawl
Squat Jump

Day 4:

Pistol Squat (Per Leg)	6/8/10
Single Leg Hip Thruster (Per Leg)	6/8/10
Split Squat (Per Leg)	6/8/10
Toe Lift	12/16/18
Bonus Move: If you feel the need to push limits add this in. Squatpocalypse: Hold a low squat at the bottom for 5 seconds, then 1 squat jump rep, hold 5 seconds then 2 squat jumps, repeated this up to 5 reps then climb back down the pyramid to 1	

Day 5:

Hand Stand Push-Up	5/7/9
Dragon Flag	4/6/8
Skin The Cat	4/6/8
Elevated Pike Press	6/8/10

The Skilled Agent:

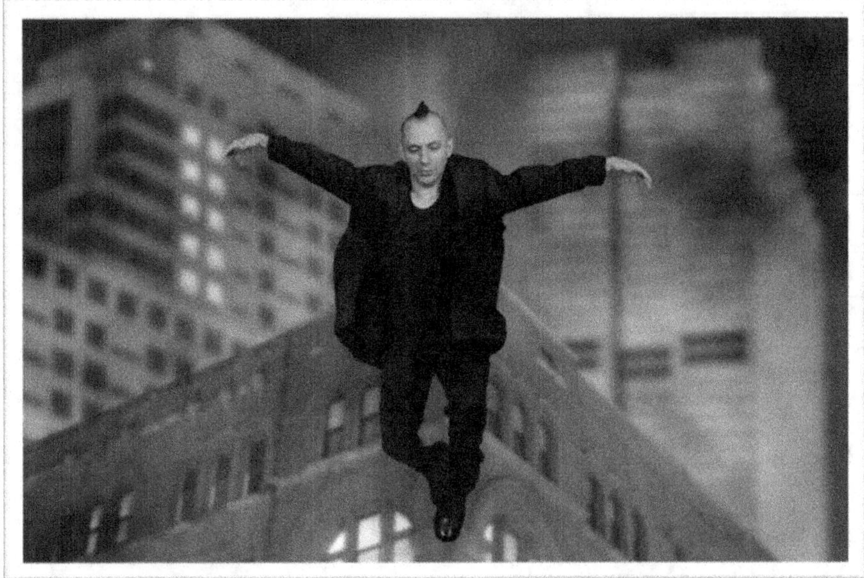

This program is very skill heavy, similar to the special agents that have to keep super humans in check. This program will have higher reps and test your endurance. Some moves will even be timed. Do you have what it takes to be an agent? Each day May bring something new to the table.

Day 1:

Each move is 30 seconds long and you will perform the most reps you can in that time. You will notice in the list there are 2 exercises separated by a "/", this means you will perform each one back to back for 30 seconds each then take a 30-60 second rest before starting the next set. Each one is 3-4 sets.

Chin-Up / Diamond Push-Up
Skin the Cat / Pike Push-Up
Pull-Up / Parallel Bar Dips
Decline Push-Up / Front Lever Swing
Pullover / L-Sit

Day 2:

Cardio Day! Perform each move for 20 seconds with a 10 second rest. 3-4 sets per move.

Squat Jump
Long Jump
Plank Toe Tap
Bear Crawl
Jumping Split Squats
Burpee

Day 3:

Each move is 4 sets with a 30-60 second rest. Any of the stunts can be switched out for another stunt you would like to achieve.

Angle Flag (Max Hold)	
Muscle Up Negative	5-8 Reps
Elbow Lever (Max Hold)	
Hand Stands	30 Second hold
Archer Push-up	12-16 reps

Day 4:

Cardio Day! Perform each move per section for 30 seconds repeating twice before you take a 30 second rest. 3 sets per section.

Plyo Push-up
Long Jump
Plank Toe Tap
Tuck Jump
Burpee
Jumping Jacks

Day 5:

Do each movement back to back for the listed rep or time count with a 60 second rest between sets.

Jumping Split Squats	30 Seconds
Full Bridge	30 Seconds
Squats	15 reps
Box Jump	12-15 reps
Archer Squat 12 reps	

Month 2:

Will push your Plyometric training. You will train to explode movement to movement while building strength. As always you can progress and regress movements as needed. There will be some days where you will do a rep count move and follow it with a timed move. Speed, accuracy and power are your allies here.

Day 1:

Each exercise section is 2-4 sets with a 30-60 second rest. Once the 2-4 sets are complete take a 1-2 minute rest before the next exercise combo.

Muscle Up 5-8 reps
L-Sit Chin-up 8-12 Reps / Mountain Climber 30 seconds
Plyometric Push-up 8-12 Reps / Jumping Jacks 30 Seconds
Commando Pull-Up 8-12 Reps / Burpee 30 Seconds
Decline Push-up 12-15 Reps / Flutter Kicks 30 Seconds
Pull-Up 10-12 reps / Bear Crawl 30 Seconds
Planche Push-Ups 12-15 Reps / Low Plank 30 Seconds

Day 2:

Each move in day 2 is 4 sets performed back to back before you take a 1-2 minute rest.

Archer Squat 12-16 reps
Alternating Single Leg Dead Lift 15 reps (per leg)
Jumping Split Squat 12-20 reps
Alternating Single Leg Hip Thrusters 12-15 (Per leg)
Wall Sit 30 Seconds
Bonus Move: If you feel the need to push limits add this in after you have finished all your sets. Squatpocalypse: Hold a low squat at the bottom for 5 seconds, then 1 squat jump rep, hold 5 seconds then 2 squat jumps, repeated this up to 5 reps then climb back down the pyramid to 1

Day 3:

Cardio day! Each is done back to back for 30 seconds each. Once the set is done rest 30 seconds and repeat for a total of 3 sets. Don't move on to the next series of movements until you finish the first 3 sets.

Mountain Climbers
Plyometric Push-Ups
Speed Skaters
High Plank & Low Plank
Burpee
Tuck Jump
Bear Crawl
Jumping Jacks

Day 4

Each move is 2-4 sets with a 30 second rest between each set. Once the sets are complete take a 2 minute rest.

Flag Training (Max Hold)
Dragon Flag 5-10 reps
Hand Stand Push-up 5-10 reps
Back Lever (Max Hold)
Elevated Pike Press Push-up 15-20 reps
Elbow Lever (Max Hold)

Day 5

Each exercise section is 2-4 sets with a 30-60 second rest. Once the 2-4 sets are complete take a 1-2 minute rest before the next exercise combo.

Squat 12-15 Reps / Long Jumps 30 seconds
Alternating Single Leg Dead Lift 12-15 (Per Leg) / Box Jump 30 Seconds
Elevated Split Squats 10-15 (Per Leg) / Jumping Split Squats 30 seconds
Single Leg Hip Thrusters 12-15 (per leg) / Bridge Hold 30 Seconds
Archer Squat 12-15 Reps (Per Leg) / Speed Skater 30 Seconds

The Energy Controller:

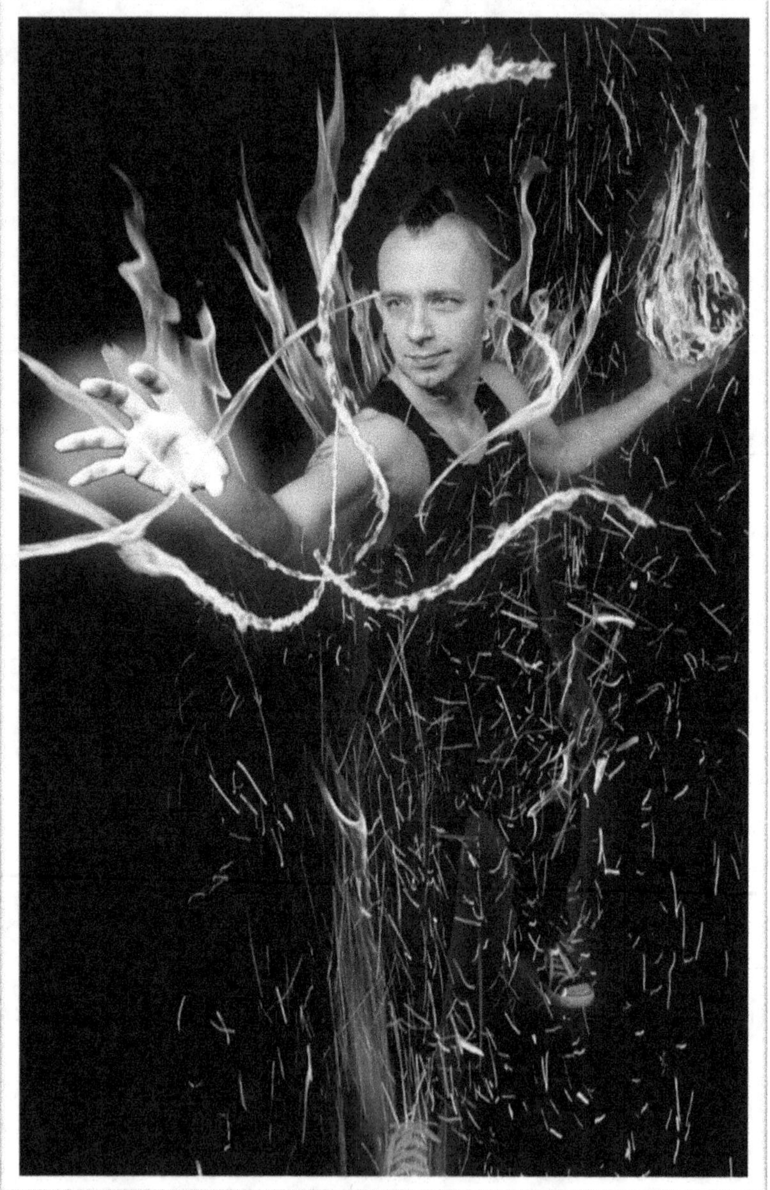

This is a balance of Strength, Skill and Cardio. This is all about alternating energy, building your cardio, strength and power with a few tricks mixed in. Build up that inner fire and give it a try.

Month 1:

It's clean and simple with little bit of both of the prior workout programs. As always focus on form and quality of movement.

Day 1:

This is your cardio day! This will be done through Tabata training. What is Tabata you ask? It is 20 seconds giving it your all followed by a 10 seconds rest. Each exercise is 4-6 rounds.

Tuck Jumps
High Plank & Low Plank
Long Jumps
Mountain Climbers
Plyometric Push-ups
Burpees
Jumping Jacks
Squat Jumps

Day 2:

Each move is maximum reps in 30 seconds for 2-4 sets and a 30-60 second rest between sets. Be sure to complete your sets before moving to the next exercise.

Pull-Up
Decline Push-up
Chin-Up
Push-Up
Parallel Bar Dips
Elevated Pike Press Push-Up

Day 3:

Cardio Day! Perform each move per section for 30 seconds repeating twice before you take a 30 second rest. 3-4 sets per section.

Jumping Split Squats
Side to Side Plank
Speed Skater
Burpee
Jumping Jacks
Bear Crawl

Day 4:

Test your tempo! You will be doing 8-10 reps with a 3/1/3 tempo at 3-4 sets. There will be a few exceptions where you will just hold a move under tension.

Pull-Ups
Push-Up
Squats
Single leg Dead Lift (Per Leg)
Pike Press
Step Ups (Per Leg)

Day 5

Each move is max reps in 30 seconds rest between sets. Be sure to complete the full circuit before taking that much needed rest. Your rest is 30-60 seconds.

Deep Squats
Push-Ups
Jumping Split Squat
Bear Crawl
Long Jumps
Body Weight Row

Month 2

This month we up the energy level, add some tricks and a bit of endurance. Is your energy level high enough?

Day 1:

Each move is 30 seconds long and you will perform the most reps you can in that time. You will notice in the list there are 2 exercises separated by a "/", this means you will perform each one back to back for 30 seconds each then take a 30-60 second rest before starting the next set. Each one is 3-4 sets.

Pull-Up / Plance Push-Up
Archer Squat / Wall Sit
Commando Pull-up / Diamond Push-Up
Squats / Jumping Split Squat
Chin-Up Hold / Push-up Hold

Day 2

Cardio Day! Perform each move per section for 30 seconds repeating twice before you take a 30 second rest. 3 sets per section.

Squat Jump
Low Plank & High Plank
Burpee
Speed Skater
Plyometric Push-Up
Knee Tucks
Jumping Split Squats
Bear Crawl

Day 3

Climb the pyramids! You will climb up and down the pyramid. Well if you see 8/10/12 after a exercise, it means set 1 is 8 reps, set 2 is 10, set 3 is 12reps, set 4 is 10 reps, set 5 is 8 reps. After each set you take a 30 second rest.

Push-Up 10/12/14
Pistol Squat 6/8/10
Pull-Up 6/8/10
Hip Thrusters 10/12/14
Dips 8/10/12
Chin-ups 6/8/10
Bonus Move: If you feel the need to push limits add this in after you have finished all your sets. Squatpocalypse: Hold a low squat at the bottom for 5 seconds, then 1 squat jump rep, hold 5 seconds then 2 squat jumps, repeated this up to 5 reps then climb back down the pyramid to 1

Day 4

Cardio Day! Perform each move per section for 30 seconds repeating twice before you take a 30 second rest. 3 sets per section.

Squat Jump
Low Plank & High Plank
Burpee
Speed Skater
Plyometric Push-Up
Knee Tucks
Jumping Split Squats
Jumping Jacks

Day 5

This is very much a trick day. A lot of it will be holding positions. You will be shocked how much holding a position can burn. Each move is 2-4 sets for a max hold.

Elbow Lever
Hand Stand
L-Sit
Back Lever
Bridge

The Super Villain!!!

This is a bonus workout, and the hardest ones you will do. You need to ask yourself, are you powerful enough to defeat it? Don't feel you need to rush into this.

5 min Run
Stretch

Round1:

Each move is 30 seconds done back to back.

Mountain Climbers
Squat Jump
Plank Toe Tap
Long Jumps
Knee Tucks
Burpees
Jumping Jacks
Speed Skaters
Pushpocalypse: Hold a Push-Up at the bottom for 5 seconds, then 1 Push-Up rep, hold 5 seconds then 2 Push-Ups, repeated this up to 5 reps then climb back down the pyramid to 1

Round 2:

Archer Squat (per leg) 15 Reps
Single Leg Deadlifts (per leg) 15 Reps
Wall Sit 1 Minute
Bonus Move: If you feel the need to push limits add this in after you have finished all your sets. Squatpocalypse: Hold a low squat at the bottom for 5 seconds, then 1 squat jump rep, hold 5 seconds then 2 squat jumps, repeated this up to 5 reps then climb back down the pyramid to 1

One arm & one leg Plank (per side) 30 seconds
Side Plank (per side) 30 Seconds
Low Plank 1 Minute
Full Bridge 30 Seconds

Round 3:

Each move is 1 minute with a 30 second rest at the end of each circuit.

5 Plyometric Push-Up / 5 Tuck Jump / 10 Mountain Climber
Burpee
5 Plyometric Push-Up / 5 Tuck Jump / 10 Mountain Climber
Burpee
Rest
5 Jump Squat / 10 Jumping Split Squats / 20 Flutter Kicks
Jumping Jacks
5 Jump Squat / 10 Jumping Split Squats / 20 Flutter Kicks
Jumping Jacks
Rest
5 Bench Dips / 5 Pike Press
Bear Crawl
5 Bench Dips / 5 Pike Press
Bear Crawl

Round 4

Each station is 30 seconds. Once each station is complete take a 30 second rest then repete.

Pull-Ups
Hand Stand
Body Weight Rows
Box Jump
Burpee

Special Thanks

I first want to thank my wife, Elisabeth, for supporting me in my passion for fitness. Without you and your advice, I may have never looked at the idea of becoming a trainer, or even considered writing a book. Being an amazing author herself, she was a huge help on this project. I absolutely love you with all of my heart.

Gerald, a.k.a. Chocolate Bear, thanks for helping me get this off the ground! Without your help editing this, I'm sure it would have been an absolute mess. Not only are you a fantastic writer, but you get me to push a little bit harder in each workout. I could not ask for a better friend in the gym.

To all my Beast Club members, thanks for tolerating all the crazy ideas I come up with for the workouts. You all keep me super motivated to keep going. We really are a true fitness family! Punch it, crunch it!

To all my clients out there, without your continued support, this book may have never happened. You all work so hard in every session and never say die. You all inspire me every day.

I also have to thank Danny and Al Kavadlo. They helped to inspire my change into the calisthenics world, and are true masters of body weight training. The time I spent training with them was an amazing experience that I try to pass to my clients.

Thank you to Café Boba, for supplying me with the needed coffee to keep me going. By far the best coffee in Grand Rapids.

Special shout out to HYLETE.com for the fantastic fitness apparel. It is by far the best fitness clothing I have ever tried. Go HYLETE Nation!

About The Author

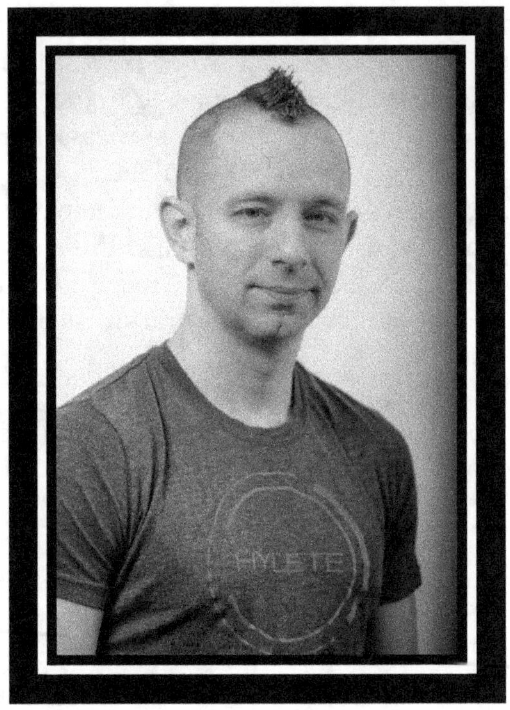

Ray Shonk is a Grand Rapids based Master Trainer, Certified Calisthenics Instructor, Tai Chi Instructor and devotes a lot of his time to improving the health and lives of his clients with a minimalist approach to fitness. Ray is also the owner of the gym Quest Fitness, and an Adjunct Professor at Grand Valley State University. In his spare time, Ray spends his time brewing beer and both console and tabletop gaming.